Alkaline Diet for Beginners

The Ultimate Plant Based Diet Guide of Alkaline Herbal Medicine for permanent weight loss, Understand pH with Anti Inflammatory Recipes Cookbook + 28 days Meal Plan

Emma Jason

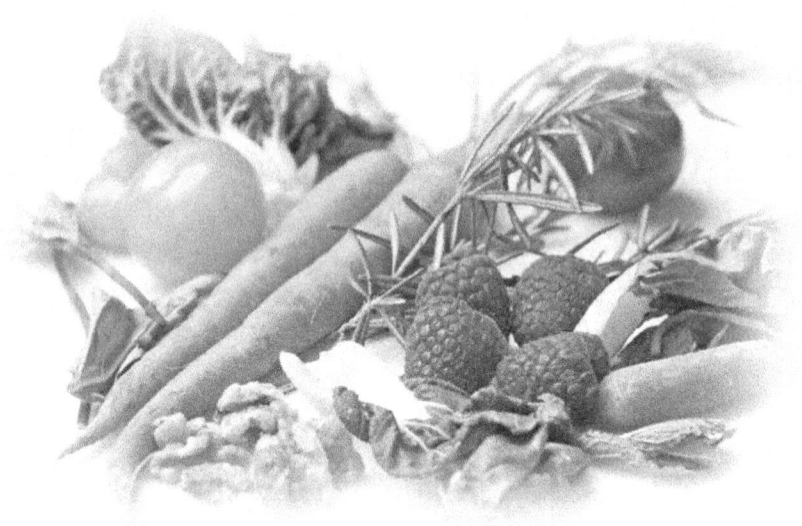

Copyright © 2019

- Emma Jason -

All rights reserved.

CONTENTS

1	What is Alkalinity? Why should I care?	Pag. 1
2	Health Risks of Inflammatory Foods and Sources	Pag. 7
3	Benefits of Alkalinity	Pag. 14
4	Week One: Meal Plan and Recipes	Pag. 36
5	Week Two: Reactivate	Pag. 43
6	Week Three: Rebuild	Pag. 51
7	Week Four: Rebalance	Pag. 59
8	Week Five: Relax	Pag. 68
9	Bonus Recipes – Snacks & Treats	Pag. 76
10	Following the Alkaline Diet	Pag. 85
11	Tasty Alkaline Recipes	Pag. 90

Introduction

Congratulations on downloading *Alkaline Diet for Beginners* and thank you for doing so.

There are plenty of books on this subject on the market, thanks again for choosing this one!
Over the past years, there have been a number of different diet plans introduced into the market. Some of these diet plans have managed to make a big impact while others faded within a few months of gaining popularity.

When it comes to weight loss, people often look for the more convenient methods to get fit rather than something that can benefit the body. If you want to lose weight, then your main motto shouldn't just be to burn fat but also to get healthy and prevent the risk of a number of diseases from occurring. You have to follow a healthy diet plan that works well on your body and mind, and also helps you stay healthy by lowering the risk of some of the most chronic illnesses which people suffer from when they do not pay attention to their health.

The reason an alkaline diet has gained so much popularity is because it focuses not only on weight loss but on decreasing the risk of diseases that are caused due to lack of nutrients and antioxidants in the body. The diet plan that was introduced in this book not only managed to prove effective when applied to your daily lifestyle, but it also turned out to be an easy diet plan to follow as soon as your body got used to it.

This detailed guide gives you hands-on information about an alkaline diet, what you need in order to follow the diet, and how it can benefit you with a few changes in your lifestyle. You will also understand why nutritionists encourage people to adapt to veganism. This guide will help you transform your mind, body, and soul!

Chapter 1 - What Is Alkalinity? Why Should I Care?

It's no hidden secret that certain foods work well on your body while others have bad side effects. But the key to understanding which food is healthy for you and what kind of food you need to avoid is important because in between a burger and a salad, there is a lot of room for you to introduce healthier options that can help your body heal from within and make you look great at the same time.

The one factor that helps you to understand how healthy you are is figuring out whether you have an alkaline body or an acidic body. If you have a high acidic level, then you need to understand how you can alkalize your body to lead a healthy lifestyle.

When you suffer from high acidic levels in your body, you are more prone to problems such as fatigue or low energy levels. Other signs of high acid levels in your body also include brittle nails and hair. It is also known to cause low bone density and osteoporosis in women which can cause multiple fractures with a simple fall. Although people do not take acidic levels in their body that seriously—but they should—it also results in heavy breathing and weight gain, which is often followed by obesity. An acidic diet can also introduce digestive issues along with diabetes. People with high acidic levels are also known to suffer from skin related problems and acne, they usually have a low immune system which means they are more susceptible to infections and allergies. These people are also at a higher risk of heart problems and cancer. If you want to stay away from these problems, it's important for you to transform your body into an alkaline body by following a healthy diet.

What Is Alkalinity?

An alkaline diet is based on the content of alkalinity in your body. Your alkalinity levels are measured by figuring out whether you have higher alkaline content or higher acidic content in your body. While the total alkalinity in your body means having a high pH level, the truth is, while pH levels are a part of an alkaline diet, it does not make up the diet completely. For instance, alkalinity in a body is measured by the amount of Alkaline substances present in the water content in your body. The normal pH level for alkalinity is anything between 0 to 14. If you have a pH level that is higher than 7, your body is neutral and if it's lower than 7, this means you have more acidic content in your system.

Anything above 7 indicates higher alkalinity levels while below 7 indicates acidic levels in the body. It is important for every person to understand the level of alkalinity in the body because a diet plan is to be based on the pH level of the individual. If your pH levels are very low, you need to make sure you stay away from acidic food and also make sure that you consume nutritious foods. Most people today have high acidic content in the system which is why focusing on an alkaline diet is something you need to consider doing. Foods such as meat and fresh dairy, eggs, grain, and alcohol all contain high acidic levels that aren't great for the body. Neutral foods are usually natural fats, sugar, and starches which also need to be avoided. An alkaline diet is basically a diet that is filled with fruits, legumes, and vegetables. These are the kind of foods you need to focus on eating to get healthy.

What Exactly Does "pH Level" Mean?

The term pH is not new and you have probably heard it numerous times in your classroom during a science class. The pH scale is basically used to measure the alkalinity or acidity in any substance where 7 is considered to be the neutral number and anything above it is alkaline where is anything below it is acidic. To measure the alkalinity or acidity in a substance, you need an aqueous solution. Human blood is aqueous because it contains high water content and this means that there is a pH level in your blood as well. This doesn't mean you can test the pH level in your blood because the pH level in your blood will not change except for when you are in a critical situation and have a life-threatening disease.

The alkaline levels in your saliva and urine, however, keep changing depending on the kind of food that you eat. This enables you to understand your cellular health. The reason this is important is because without monitoring the cellular level, you will not manage to figure out whether you are healthy or not.

While the pH levels in your blood usually clock under 7, the levels in urine could go as low as 3. To begin following a healthy alkaline diet, you need to understand how long your levels of alkalinity are. This will help you figure out what needs to be changed and how you have to make the changes.

The reason monitoring your pH levels is important is because when it goes considerably low, your body turns acidic and you could even suffer from something known as chronic low-grade acidosis. This is normally caused when there is a high consumption of acidic foods that impact your body and results in low calcium, potassium, magnesium, and mineral levels in your body.

Research has proven that following an alkaline diet can help reduce multiple health-related problems and aid in effective weight loss. This is why it's important for you to understand how the pH levels in your body impact your overall health.

What Is the Alkaline Diet?

An alkaline diet is a diet that helps lower the acidic levels in your body by maintaining the pH balance. Therefore, you lose weight and get healthier, lowering the risk of multiple diseases. This diet had gained a lot of popularity when nutritionists openly spoke about how effective it is and how incorporating the diet plan into your daily routine can help you lead a longer and more fruitful life.

Figuring out an alkaline diet could cause a lot of confusion because this diet may seem very complicated when you take a glance. In theory, an alkaline diet is a diet that helps lower your body's acidic levels. This may seem like a bit tough to understand but when you start consuming fruits that have higher alkaline content and lower acidic content, it is obvious that your body starts healing. This will make it come closer to a healthy alkaline level rather than an acidic one. There are tons of food that reduce a lot of acid in your body and people are so used to consuming these foods on a regular basis, they don't realize what's affecting their body. Following a regular diet plan may seem like the perfect solution because it reflects on your weighing scale and you even notice that you have lost a few pounds. However, that doesn't necessarily mean you are getting any healthier. If you want to stay healthy, you have to lower the risk of diseases in your system and keep your vital organs functioning effectively. That's what an alkaline diet does to you which is why once people understand how effective the diet plan is, they start adapting towards leading an alkaline lifestyle and avoiding foods that have high acidic content.

Testing Yourself for Acidity

Once you have decided you want to follow the alkaline diet, you need to start planning the small changes in your lifestyle one step at a time. Taking a plunge into the first diet plan you see is not the ideal solution because everybody is different and for you to make the most out of this diet plan, you need to understand your pH level before you move forward. To do this, you need to test your acid levels and see just how high the acidic level is.

Testing for acidic levels in your body is very simple. You need to get a pH test paper. This paper tests the acid and alkaline levels of any liquid and you can either use urine or saliva to test your acidic levels. However, it is highly recommended that you test it with the first urine you collect in the morning after at least 6 hours of uninterrupted sleep. To do the test, all you need to do is take a strip of the paper and dip it into a cup of urine you have accumulated or urinate directly on the paper. If you are not comfortable urinating, you can then spit on the paper as soon as you get up in the morning.

When you purchase the pH paper, it comes with a color chart to help you figure out just how acidic or basic your body is. The colors usually range from yellow to blue and they have numbers written by their side. As mentioned earlier, if you are below seven, it means you are on the acidic side but if you are above 7, you are healthy.

There is more sense to purchase the pH test paper and use it every now and then. The reason being once you incorporate the diet plan you will manage to measure results on a regular basis and this helps keep your motivation levels high.

Signs Your Body Is Too Acidic

While it may be easy to get pH testing paper from various shopping websites all over the internet, in case you haven't managed to find this test strip yet, you can always look out for the early warning signs. These signs will tell if your body is too acidic and you need to take charge for you to live a healthy life.

1. One of the major signs that your body is too acidic is when you start feeling too tired even if you've rested for over 8 hours every night. People who have a high acid content in their system tend to feel tired and low on energy even with enough rest.

2. High acidic levels in your body also make you feel sad and depressed most of the time. Even it is a reason to celebrate and you still can't feel genuinely happy, this could be a sign that you have high acidic levels in your body.

3. People who suffer from high acidic levels also tend to get irritable for no apparent reason and they snap very easily. If you are told that you are snappy or irritable, this could be because you have high acidic levels.

4. Another common sign that you have high acidic levels is the inability to focus effectively on your task. If you find it difficult to get your mind in one place and get a job done effectively, this is another sign that your acidic levels are high and it needs to be brought down under control.

5. Low immunity levels and the susceptibility to infections such as cold and flu is another common sign of a high acidic level.

6. People who also suffer from skin problems and dry skin, even during warmer months of the year, could have a high acidic level.

7. Hormonal imbalance is another sign that you need to be on the lookout for.

8. Another common problem involves digestive issues which could be a combination of constipation along with diarrhea.

9. Shortness of breath, chronic pain, sensitivity in teeth and gums and a stiff neck are also common signs that your body is too acidic and you need to do something to change it.

These are some of the early signs and the sooner you identify them, the better it is because you will manage to shift towards a healthy diet plan.

Chapter 2 - Health Risks of Inflammatory Foods and Sources

There are various situations and conditions that contribute to inflammation. These conditions exert physiological stress on the body, lead to high levels of sugar, and inhibit lipid digestion.

Conditions that contribute to inflammation include:

Foods we consume: Diet is by far the greatest contributor to inflammation and there are many contributing foods that we might consume. Certainly, sugary foods will increase the chances of inflammation in our blood vessels. The process through which foods causes inflammation begins in the jejunum, as our food is digested. The more foods we have within the intestines that the body views as invading rivals, the more toxins that enter our bloodstream. When your body senses foreign substances in the digestive system, it sends a message to the protective system of the body and there is an attack, a battle. As a protective measure, the system releases its counter attacking cells such as lymphocytes. The entire body strives to block these invaders from entering into every cell and this leads to inflammation in the overall bloodstream. Therefore, eating unhealthily is a great contributor to inflammation and severe infections.

Inability to remove the cause of inflammation: Further, inflammation in your bloodstream prevents sufficient sugar from getting into the brain cells. Since brain cells need sugar to function, you end up needing more glucose and feeding into more sugary foodstuff to get glucose. The ultimate result of this is chronic inflammation.

Eating habits: Poor eating habits like hasty eating stresses the body and at times like this the body is unable to absorb nutrients needed to keep you healthy.

Stress: A strong link exists between stress and anxiety and instances and aggravation of inflammation, yet the crucial central nervous system is one of the most overlooked elements in the body's inflammatory process. It is good to understand that CNS triggers the immune process to respond to tissue injury or infection. Stress and anxiety activate the inflammatory pathway and can also develop the body's urge to consume those inflammatory foods even when we are not hungry. Stress feeding, with calorie-filled and nutrient-poor foods furthers the cycle and endorses the condition of being overweight, which is known to cause inflammation.

Socio-economic environment: The environment that you live in may influence your lifestyle, which will in turn influence your immune system. Your community may make you believe that you have to eat something, even though it feels like your body does not work well with it. Income will impact your ability to sustain all of your needs; You may not be able to afford a costly alkaline diet. Unfortunately, you may not even know which low-cost foods are also part of the alkaline diet.

Why Chronic Inflammation Is a Risk to Your Health?

Scientists argue that when the inflammatory cells stay for long in the blood, they lead to a condition known as plague. The plague is perceived by the immune system as a foreign invader in the body and as such, your system strives to prevent the plague within the blood vessels from getting inside arteries. Over time, the plague may become wobbly and rupture, forming a lump that blocks sufficient blood flow throughout the body. Consequently, this leads to the condition of stroke or heart attack, otherwise known as cardiovascular disease (CVD) and among the highest cause of mortality in the developed nations.

Cancer
Usually, chronic inflammation that lasts and persists within the body leads to damage of the Deoxyribonucleic acid (DNA), and which ultimately causes tumor development.

Type 2 Diabetes
Being unable to produce sufficient insulin, a chemical responsible for maintaining sustainable levels of blood sugar, is a characteristic inherent in Diabetes victims. Scientists have found out that people whose blood sugar is unregulated have higher inflammation levels than people without. The implication of this is that low-grade inflammation alters the action of insulin in the body, and hence can cause Type 2 Diabetes.

Arthritis
Arthritis is a major inflammation-related condition. Arthritis is described as an inflammation of the joints. While inflammation is connected to rheumatoid arthritis and gouty arthritis, some types of arthritis like osteoarthritis are not caused by inflammation.

Treatment for Chronic Inflammation
As previously mentioned, inflammation is part of the healing process, in the case of infected tissues. However, sometimes reducing inflammation is also helpful. There are alkaline drugs, herbs, and supplements on the market today.

Although to date, no drug has been found whose direct function is to cure chronic inflammation, there are over the counter medicines that can treat and help manage the symptoms of acute or chronic inflammation. These medicines include aspirin and ibuprofen which are classed within the category of non-fat insoluble drugs. They work by destroying the substances that cause inflammation and can provide relief from the pain and fever associated with inflammation. However, when taken over a long period of time, these drugs can lead to the development of other infections which manifest as severe side effects so these drugs should be avoided as a long-term solution.

For cases of chronic inflammation, medicines which include ingredients like prednisone and cortisone are prescribed to stop inflammation. They contain the steroid hormone which combats inflammation. The consumption of these drugs come with the potential for negative side effects like fluid retention and weight gain. Other drugs may come in the form of salves, often used to treat inflammation in the lungs, bowels, eyes, and skin.

Devil's claw is a recognized dietary supplement that acts as an effective suppressor of severe inflammation, although the evidence available today of their usage is limited. Besides this, herbs such as Hyssop oils, Turmeric, Ginger and Cannabis are known to inhibit the development of inflammatory reactions within the body system. They have been used in the concept of disease treatment and prevention long into the history of our human civilization and they have been effective in relieving arthritis pains and soreness in the lungs, among other illnesses. Apart from Cannabis, herbs are easily available in most areas. In the case of the Cannabis herb, the legislation around its possession and use varies from place to place.

Overall, alkaline diets and positive changes in lifestyle are among the most efficient and fulfilling treatments for inflammation. Not only does a diet that consists of alkaline foods suppress our levels of inflammation, this diet also helps to prevent inflammation. Not surprisingly, alkaline diets have become a common cure for chronic inflammation.

Alkaline Water
When you adopt an alkaline diet, the one thing you need to learn is to prepare alkaline water. Alkaline water is nothing but water that has its alkaline levels boosted up to benefit you better. This water works

wonders on your body and it helps to keep you healthy. One of the best things about alkaline water is that it has more hydrating properties in comparison to normal water, which means if you exercise or your body requires more water, the molecules in alkaline water can help rehydrate your body a lot faster than normal water.

Since the alkaline levels in the water are increased, it also boosts your immunity system and helps to fight off bacteria and infections more effectively. Regular consumption of alkaline water can work well to enhance your diet and take off all environmental toxins including stress. Unlike normal water, alkaline water contains a lot of magnesium and calcium and this contributes towards healthy bones. Since it has high antioxidant content, it also takes care of free radical cells and lowers the risk of cancer. Apart from fighting off diseases, alkaline water can also reverse the signs of aging and give you beautiful skin and hair. One of the best things about alkaline water is that it helps to lower the acidity in the system and it keeps your stomach and gastrointestinal tract healthy.

Green Drinks / Smoothies
Greens have become an integral part of your diet and they should be included in every form possible. While we have seen the benefits of including raw greens in your daily diet, including green drinks or green smoothies can also benefit your physical health in a number of ways. Here are a few benefits of green smoothies that you probably didn't know about.

- **Healthy Mentality**
  Green smoothies help you have a very positive and healthy frame of mind. The human mind is very difficult to train and it thrives on consistency. This means that if you start one particular habit that is healthy, your mind will start encouraging you to start another healthy habit. Try adding kale to your smoothie and see the mental change that it

brings about. You will then want to take up a Yoga class that you have always wanted to try or go for a run on a daily basis when your smoothie intake is green.

- **Reduce Unhealthy Cravings**
  When you start consuming a green smoothie on a daily basis, you will feel nourished and not crave for unhealthy sweets or foods. This can again be tied to the mental frame of mind where your mind will want to continue the healthy transformation and encourage you to eat healthy snacks. Green smoothies are a great way to cut down on the binge eating and reduce the number of unhealthy snacks that you consume daily.

- **Glowing Skin**
  Since greens are rich in antioxidants, it does have a positive impact on your skin and you will see that your skin is hydrated and even the signs of aging have reduced.

- **Healthy Heart**
  As you are already aware, greens are rich in antioxidants and they help to lower your cholesterol and keep away heart-related problems.

- **Immunity Boost**
  Greens help boost your immune system and it will keep you away from illnesses for as long as you are consuming them. Consuming a green smoothie on a daily basis will keep you healthier than others who do not.

- **Better Digestion**
  Since smoothies utilize whole veggies, there is a lot of fiber that you receive and this will help improve your digestion.

- **Nutrient Absorption**

When you consume smoothies daily, you will receive a lot of nutrients from vegetables such as spinach, kale, and lettuce.

- **Better Energy**
  When you start absorbing a lot of nutrients every day, your energy levels will be very high and you will feel very invigorated.

Other Foods

It's confusing to differentiate between foods that are highly acidic or alkaline, and that's the reason why people who just start out on an alkaline diet often end up eating the wrong kind of food. Just because something is vegan doesn't necessarily mean it is alkaline and it could benefit you. When you are on an alkaline diet, you should try and include alkaline fruits, nuts, legumes, and veggies. You should try to avoid foods that have high acid levels such as meat, poultry, fish, dairy, eggs, grains, and alcohol.

However, make sure that the fruits, nuts, legumes, and vegetables you include in your diet are highly alkaline and can promote the benefits of following the diet. There are some amazing alkaline foods that you should try to incorporate in your diet apart from the regular list that you will come across. These include soy products such as soya bean, miso, tofu, and tempeh. You can also look for unsweetened varieties of yogurt and curd as well as milk. Although some diets suggest that potatoes need to be avoided, you can most definitely include a small portion of potatoes when you are on an alkaline diet. You can also try to use as many herbs and spices to add flavor to your food.

Chapter 3 - Benefits of Alkalinity

An alkaline diet is all about increasing the alkalinity in your body to help you lead a healthy and long life that's disease free. This diet plan has been making waves in the market because of the effectiveness that it has to offer and more and more people are now planning to get used to the diet plan.

One of the major reasons why the alkaline diet has gained so much popularity is because it helps people get slim; however, that's not the only thing that alkalinity can help you with. Once you understand how alkalinity works and what it does to your body, you will never want to switch back to a diet plan that contains a high acid content.

Protects Bone Density and Muscle Mass
Research has proven that high acid content in your body can affect your bones as well as your muscles. The reason it is important for you to focus on alkaline meals is because it increases the mineral intake in your body and focuses on better bone structure, resulting in lesser brittle bones. The acid content in your body is responsible for bone problems including joint pain and arthritis. When you lower the acid contents in your body, it gets easier for your bones to become stronger and absorb the healthy minerals that contribute towards better bone health. An alkaline diet focuses on increasing the production of vitamin D absorption in the bone and this is responsible for keeping your bones healthy. It also helps in the production of growth hormone and in ensuring that your body gets more strength from the minerals consumed. This helps effectively increase muscle mass and strength.

By increasing the alkalinity in your body, not only do you get better bones and better muscle strength but your endurance increases and you manage to exercise more effectively. This is vital for your overall health and it helps to keep away a number of bone-related diseases. When you have strong muscles, your body stays firmer and you age more gracefully.

Lowers Risk for Hypertension and Stroke

Following an alkaline diet has a lot of anti-aging effects on the body. Apart from helping to protect muscle mass, it also decreases inflammation in the body and this works well to relieve a lot of stress and enhances cardiovascular health. People who follow an alkaline diet are less prone to hypertension and cholesterol. One of the leading causes of stroke is high cholesterol levels and blood clots caused by this cholesterol content. When you start an alkaline diet, your cholesterol level falls into place and it also helps to regulate blood pressure which is responsible for hypertension.

When you relieve stress, you start leading a healthy life not only physically but mentally as well. Stress is directly related to memory loss and a number of brain-related illnesses including Alzheimer's disease and Dementia. When you consume an alkaline based diet, you lower the risk of these diseases and also prevent the risk of a heart attack and high blood pressure.

Alkaline-based diets also work really well on your vital organs including your kidneys. Kidney stones can be excruciatingly painful. One of the major causes of kidney stone is the acid content in your body and when this content is reduced, you lower the risk.

Lowers Chronic Pain and Inflammation

It's no secret that some women suffer from severe menstrual cramps during their menstruation while others manage to handle it more effectively. The leading cause of cramps during menstruation is high acid levels in the body. When you begin following an alkaline based diet, you reduce the risk of suffering from painful cramps because it helps soothe the muscles and relax them.

Alkalinity also helps prevent chronic back pain, muscle spasms, headache, inflammation, and joint pains. By simply reducing the acid levels in your body, you can keep a number of these problems at bay. When your body is healthier, you have more energy and you are able to get a lot more done during the day. It is important for you to have relaxed muscles and keep away inflammation and chronic pain to start leading a healthy lifestyle. This is where alkalinity comes into the picture and this is why it's so important.

Boosts Vitamin Absorption and Prevents Magnesium Deficiency

Magnesium deficiency is highly underrated and people don't understand the importance of getting adequate magnesium in your body. When you are unable to provide your body with the right amount, a lot of enzymes in your system begin dysfunctioning and it's not possible for your body to carry out its regular processes effectively. Lack of magnesium is one of the main causes of heart diseases and muscle spasms. It is also responsible for headache, sleep anxiety, and insomnia. When your magnesium levels are optimum, it also helps in activating Vitamin D and boosts the absorption of this vitamin into your bones for healthier and stronger bones. Magnesium also works well with other vitamins and helps the body get the benefits of those vitamins by absorbing it more effectively.

Helps Improve Immune Functionality and Cancer Protection

One of the major benefits of alkalinity is that it helps oxidize your body more effectively and dispose of waste material faster. Apart from helping boost your metabolism level, it also strengthens the immune system to get rid of the dirty toxins on a regular basis. When you have a stronger immune system, your body manages to fight off bacteria and infections better. An alkaline diet contains high antioxidant properties responsible for fighting off the free radical cells mainly responsible for cancer cells growing in the system. An alkaline diet can help reduce the risk of cancer by killing these cells.

People who have multiple health problems should move to an alkaline based diet because not only does this help your body cope with medical treatments, but it also helps you respond to the treatment better and encourages healing. Research has proven that chemotherapy works better when your pH levels are well balanced.

Can Help You Maintain a Healthy Weight

One of the major reasons why an alkaline-based diet has gained so much popularity is because it helps burn fat and bring you back in shape. Unlike other diet plans that promise you effective results in just 30 days, this diet plan helps you to stay fit and active and helps you to fight off diseases which are most important. When you shift from an acid-based diet to an alkaline diet, you automatically start lowering the amount of calories you consume and this helps your body burn fat faster. It also helps your body to get stronger and it gives you more energy.

Best Alkaline Foods

A common misconception about an alkaline based diet is that you need to simply shift to a vegan lifestyle and you start getting healthy. Although vegan food is good, in order for you to increase the alkalinity in your body, you have to consume foods that have high alkaline content.

Fresh Fruits and Vegetables

When you are following an effective alkaline diet, it means including as much fruit and vegetable as possible. These fruits and vegetables work really well to balance the pH level in your body, making you healthier and more active. There is a variety you can purchase from the market but not all of these are great for alkaline diets. Here is a list of the most effective fruits and vegetables you should try to incorporate in your diet plan to increase alkaline levels in the body.

Avocado

Avocado is an amazing fruit when you are on an alkaline diet. Not only does it help reduce acidic levels in your body, but it also provides you with a lot of nutrients such as vitamin B, E, C and K. It also has a high content of potassium and copper along with monounsaturated healthy fats. Avocado contains dietary fiber which is great for your metabolism and also works well to aid weight loss because it helps you feel fuller for longer.

Broccoli
Although this vegetable isn't a favorite for a lot of people, including broccoli in your meals can give you a number of benefits. Broccoli is probably one of the rare vegetables that are packed with nutrients that include Vitamin B6, K, and C. It also has a high content of magnesium folate, Phosphorus Selenium, and potassium that help diminish the acidic effects in your body and boost the alkaline content. It is always best to eat the vegetable raw.

Celery
Celery has high Vitamin B and C content. It also offers alkaline and antioxidant properties which help to enhance cardiovascular functionality. Celery helps to fight oxidative stress, keeping your body relieved and enhancing muscle mass as well as relaxing your muscles and your brain. Celery is a great vegetable to prevent dehydration since it has a lot of water content. The vegetable also has a lot of folate and potassium.

Cucumber
If there is one vegetable that can keep you hydrated all day long, it's cucumber. Cucumber contains 96% water that helps increase your alkaline level and also releases your body of all the dirty toxins built up inside. Cucumbers are a rich source of vitamins and minerals such as Silicon, potassium, and magnesium.

Lemon

Although a lot of people believe that lemon has high acidic content, the truth is it is actually alkaline that's inside the lemon. This citrus fruit works wonders on your digestive system and also help in better nutrition absorption. When making a salad, squeeze a generous amount of lemon on your meal and you will manage to absorb the nutrients in the salad a lot better. Vitamin C also helps to boost your immunity and protect your body against a number of illnesses because of the high Vitamin C content in it.

Peppers

Peppers are a great way to add flavor and color to your food. Whether you purchase green, yellow, or red bell peppers, they all have equal health benefits and provide you with a lot of Vitamin C and A. Peppers are also a great source of dietary fiber. Peppers contain a lot of antioxidants which help protect your body against cancer free radical cells.

Spinach

If Popeye taught you anything, it's to eat as much spinach as you can. This leafy vegetable has a high nutrient profile and it provides your body with vitamins A, C, B2, and K. It also contains high levels of iron, magnesium, manganese, folate, as well as iron. Another great benefit of eating spinach is that it helps improve the alkaline-acid ratio in your body.

All Raw Foods

The alkaline diet works best when you include raw food in your diet. The diet works well because you have kept the complete nutrition intact that the food has to offer. Whether it is in the shape of a salad, a soup, or a smoothie, incorporate as much raw food as you can to boost your alkalinity and get healthier than ever before. One of the major reasons why you need to eat your food raw is because it's in the natural form and natural ingredients work best with alkalinity. When you cook your ingredients, it tends to lose a lot of the nutrients and it will not benefit your body as much as you would like it to. Some fruits and leafy vegetables have a high antioxidant content that are lost the minute it hits the heat. This is why you should try to incorporate as much raw food as possible in your diet. The best part about an alkaline diet is that you have a wide range of fruits and vegetables to choose from and these are best enjoyed raw.

Alkaline Herbs and Supplements

If you thought going on an alkaline diet means you need to avoid adding flavor to your food, then you couldn't be more wrong. As long as it's healthy, you can use all kinds of spices and herbs to flavor your meal. The best part of an alkaline diet is you will find a wide range of herbs and supplements that you can use in your favor.

Herbs

Following an alkaline diet could get difficult because of the number of food items you need to stop consuming especially when you are used to being a non-vegetarian. However, when you look at the bright side of things, there are tons of herbs you can add to your meals to add flavor and make it more palatable. Here are some herbs that not only add flavor but also work wonders with your health.

- **Cayenne Pepper**

Cayenne peppers add an amazing flavor to your food and while this is a pungent herb, it seems to be gaining a lot of popularity due to its taste. It has a lot of alkaline properties that work well to treat headaches and arthritis. It is also known to help reduce the signs of cancer. Cayenne pepper has also been associated with weight loss.

- **Dandelion Greens**

Dandelion Greens can add amazing flavor to your salad and you can also use it to make herbal tea. It has high alkaline properties and is known to treat kidney stones effectively.

- **Turmeric**

The bright yellow spice which is known to favor a number of curries has amazing properties and is also known to treat arthritis, cancer, and diabetes. It has a lot of medicinal properties and has been used by people for decades. If you can get your hands on fresh turmeric (the ones that look like ginger), you can use it not just to flavor your food but to make pickle and consume it with your meals. This works well to control your sugar levels and keep your bones healthy.

- **Garlic**

The amazing antifungal and antibiotic properties that garlic has can help heal your body from within very effectively. Garlic is an amazing antioxidant and it also helps fight parasites in the body and making you stronger. Garlic is also known to be great for the heart and has high alkaline properties.

Supplements

Although there are a number of foods that can help increase the levels of alkaline in your body, sometimes you need a little assistance and, in this situation, supplements play a vital role. Here are a few supplements that you may be advised to take depending on the kind of diet plan you follow.

- **Potassium Citrate and Magnesium Citrate**

  For alkalization to kick in, you need to have high levels of potassium and magnesium citrate. This is so that it lowers the amount of urine that is passed out of your body and also helps to enhance bone density and reduce the risk of brittle bones and fractures.

- **Calcium**

  Calcium is an important supplement that you may want to start consuming when on an alkaline diet not only because it keeps your bones healthy, but it also helps in reducing hypertension.

- **Glutamine**
  This supplement provides the body with amino acids which are necessary to lower the acidic levels and also helps to keep your kidney functioning effectively.

- **Vitamin D**
  Without adequate vitamin D in your body, it will not manage to absorb calcium and magnesium effectively. This is why it's also important you consume this supplement through the food you are eating.

Anti-Alkaline Foods and Habits

Starting off your alkaline diet might be tougher than you expected because of the various changes you need to make in your lifestyle in order to lower the acid levels and bring up your alkaline levels to an optimum level. There are various things that happen to your body when the acid levels are high and to bring this in control, it's necessary that you change your eating habits. The reason an alkaline diet is so necessary is because it helps reduce inflammation in the body which is one of the leading causes of various diseases including arthritis, diabetes, and cancer. It also causes chronic fatigue, irritability, unnecessary food cravings, and digestive problems. If you want to lead a healthy life and look great, it's important to address the root cause of all these problems which is high acid content in the body.

Once you bring your pH levels to the optimum level, it benefits you a great deal and you start feeling better about yourself. Not only do you manage to lose weight, but you also feel more energetic and you drive away a number of illnesses. If you are diabetic, you will notice your sugar levels are in control and you will manage to get more done in a day because you simply feel great.

To follow a healthy alkaline diet, make sure you avoid meat and fish, food that contains any dairy product, eggs, alcohol, or nicotine and drugs, as well as refined grains of processed food. You should also try and stay away from any food items that have high sugar content as this isn't good for your body. Packaged cereal is also something you may want to avoid along with fast food. These foods have high acid levels and are not recommended during an alkaline diet.

Although alkaline diets do not recommend it, you avoid roasted nuts and seeds, tofu, tempeh, and soya bean in any form. It is highly recommended that you control eating these food items and never eat them more than twice a week. Food items that include vinegar or apple cider can be included in your diet more often since it's high alkaline. Avoid processed chocolates and dry fruits which have sugar added to it. Readymade salad dressings should also be limited since they are not great to consume on a daily basis.

If you want to train your mind to eat healthily, you need to take small steps and start with a few changes at a time so that your body gets used to it. If you are a hardcore non-vegetarian and you eat meat five to six times a week, do not give it up completely but instead decrease the size and limit your intake until you are comfortable giving it up and following an alkaline diet. An important rule to follow when choosing a diet plan, irrespective of which one it is, is to not force your body and make sure that whatever you plan on doing, your body is fine with it.

High-Sodium Foods: Processed Foods
Processed foods are unhealthy, which is why they should be avoided completely whether or not you are on an alkaline diet. One of the major reasons why they are so bad is because most processed foods are loaded with sugar that adds unnecessary calories in your body and doesn't benefit

you in any way. Processed foods contain no fiber content which means they affect your digestion and they don't work well for your metabolism levels as well. Processed foods are highly addictive and this means that once you get hooked on to eating these foods, it is going to be difficult for you to stop. They are known to cause mood swings and they can lead to irritability and sometimes put you in a depressed state of mind. Most processed foods have high sodium content that is not healthy for you and is known to increase blood pressure. Processed food also interferes with your sleeping habits, making it difficult for you to get sound sleep. Since these food items are made to last long, they are loaded with preservatives which could take a longer time to digest and eventually lead to a lot of weight gain.

Cold Cuts and Conventional Meats
When you lead a hectic life, cold cuts could work as a savior as they are just sitting in the freezer waiting for you to pull out and make a sandwich or a quick meal out of it. What most people don't realize is cold cuts are generally the main cause of health-related problems including high blood pressure, obesity, and high cholesterol. Cold cuts are cured meats which are preserved either by salting or smoking, and in some cases are preserved with chemicals such as sodium nitrate, all of which have high health risks. They have a lot of unnecessary calories and should be avoided if you want to lead a healthy life. Reducing the number of cold cuts in your diet can help reduce the risk of cancer, according to the World Health Organization.

Processed Cereals
Processed cereals are easy to use for people who are always on the rush. The problem with processed cereal is that it either has a lot of sugar content or the ones that are low on sugar levels contain artificial sweeteners, both of which are highly acidic for the body. These contain toxic ingredients that only destroy your body over time and don't benefit you in any way. They do not have any nutrients and only keep you full for a couple of hours before your body starts craving for more junk food.

Eggs

Eggs are a controversial subject when it comes to following an alkaline diet because an alkaline diet asks you to avoid it completely. While they usually say that an egg is healthy, the truth is consuming it may not be as beneficial as you imagine them to be. While they are high in protein content, eggs also contain a lot of cholesterol which is not great for your system and can increase the risk of a heart attack and clogged arteries. High cholesterol levels are often linked with liver cancer which is why you may want to avoid eating an egg if you want to keep your liver healthy. It is also believed that eggs contain chlorine, a compound that is highly toxic and starts growing in the gut of the person thereby increasing the risk of various health conditions. Eggs are also known to be highly acidic which affects the alkaline levels in your body and causes multiple health issues.

Caffeinated Drinks and Alcohol

Drinks that have high caffeine form bubbles in the stomach causing it to expand and giving you the feeling of bloatedness. This is an uncomfortable feeling not only because you start feeling sick but also because it affects your digestive system. Foods that contain caffeine and aerated drinks are highly acidic and should be avoided when you are on an alkaline diet and trying to get healthy. These drinks are also often loaded with a lot of sugar which adds unnecessary calories to your diet.

When you start an alkaline diet, the first thing you need to get out of your list is alcohol because alcohol is highly acidic and it could increase the amount of gastric acid in your system. The worst part about alcohol is people start consuming it with a number of carbonated drinks that multiplies the problem and creates uncomfortable situations for your body. Alcohol is not good for your liver and people who drink are more prone to liver-related issues including enlargement of the liver and cirrhosis of the liver, both of which can be avoided by cutting down on your alcohol consumption. Let's not forget, alcohol and caffeine interfere with your pH balance and push you more towards the acidic side.

Oats and Whole Wheat Products

Oats and whole wheat may sound amazing to consume when you are on a diet but these are also food products you may want to avoid when you switch to an alkaline diet. Although oats and whole wheat are healthy, the problem with both these items is that they are complex carbohydrates that take a longer time to break down in your body, thereby making it difficult for the body to digest the food. This increases the acid levels in your system and makes it difficult to maintain a healthy pH balance when you are trying to get your body's alkaline levels high.

Milk
As a child, you were told you should drink a glass of milk to make your bones healthy. The truth however, is that cow's milk actually takes off the Calcium from your bones. While calcium is an amazing acid neutralizer, milk isn't and it tends to add more acid to your body than you can imagine. This means every time you drink a glass of milk, your body is drained of the calcium content thereby increasing the acid levels. Several researchers have proven that milk can lead to prostate cancer which is why people should switch to soy milk instead. Your body needs a lot of time to digest milk and if it isn't digested properly, it could lead to bloating, diarrhea, and cramps that could make you uncomfortable.

Milk also has a lot of cholesterol and regular consumption can increase your cholesterol levels quite a bit. Research has proven that people who consume more milk are more prone to ovarian cancer. If you have heard that you should only use antibiotics when prescribed by a doctor and always complete the dosage so that your body does not start building a resistance towards the medication, you may want to stay off milk because cow's milk contains antibiotics and they start entering your system the minute you drink it and creates an anti drug-resistant atmosphere in your body. You won't even know what drugs you are resistant to because you haven't consumed them directly. Milk is often linked to weight gain and people who drink milk on a regular basis tend to add more weight in comparison to those who don't. You can substitute milk with soy-based milk products that are healthy and more alkaline in nature.

Peanuts and Walnuts
While an alkaline diet asks you to consume nuts on a regular basis, you need to stay away from peanuts and walnuts for a reason. Both peanuts and walnuts are known to increase the acid levels in your body and this is why you may want to stay away from them. These nuts interfere with the pH balance in your body and make it difficult

for you to come to the level of alkalinity that you wish. These nuts are also known to create multiple health issues including congestion and interference in the detoxification process during an alkaline diet. Unlike most of the other nuts that help you to lose weight, peanuts and walnuts are generally associated with weight gain which is why you may want to stay away from them during your alkaline diet.

Pasta, Rice, Bread and Packaged Grain Products
If you are starting an alkaline diet, the one thing you have to lay off is your pasta, rice, and bread for a reason. They are known to cause the number of dietary issues because of the heavy carbohydrates and starch content that they have. These increase the acidity in your body and are known to cause gas and heat burn along with bloating. They are also known to release complex sugars which are difficult to digest and gets accumulated as fat in your body.

The Kind of Habits That Can Cause Acidity in Your Body

If you are going on an alkaline diet, it isn't just about what you eat but also what you need to avoid to get healthy. If you want your alkaline diet to go well, you need to identify the biggest offender of the diet and stay as far away from them as possible.

Alcohol and Drugs
We have already understood that alcohol has high acid content which is why you should avoid it. Alcohol has many underlying effects as well such as causing depression and stress on a person. The problem with alcohol is that it's addictive and just like drugs, it could make you lethargic and lazy. Drugs are also high in acid content and when you start consuming drugs or start smoking on a regular basis, you are increasing the acid content in your body. If you want to follow a healthy alkaline diet, you need to cut off the alcohol and stop smoking or stop consuming drugs in any form.

High Caffeine Intake

Caffeine in any form should be avoided because it interferes with the functionality of your body and increases your heart rate unnecessarily. Caffeine also has high acid content along with a lot of unwanted sugar which results in weight gain. Consuming too many caffeine products will interfere with your sleeping habit and this causes stress as well as improper functionality of the organs.

Antibiotic Overuse

When you start popping pills unnecessarily, this does not benefit you in any way and it makes your body so used to those medicines that they won't work even when you actually have an infection that needs to be treated. These infections are known as drug-resistant infections and they are only caused when you abuse antibiotics and consume them over your recommended amount. Too much antibiotics also result in acid reflux and high acidity levels in your body which has a number of side effects and affects your alkaline diet.

Artificial Sweeteners

Artificial sweeteners are highly acidic and interfere with the process of an alkaline diet. If you want to stay healthy, you have to learn to avoid your cravings for sweets and this includes artificial sweeteners. The best artificial sweeteners are registered as low as 2.5 on a pH balance scale meaning that they are extremely acidic. If you continue using artificial sweeteners in your diet, you will not manage to bring your pH balance to the alkaline level you desire and the diet will not work as planned.

Chronic Stress

High stress level usually results in acidity and acid reflux, which is why it's important for you to learn how to relax and calm your body before you take on an alkaline diet. If you suffer from serious stress, it is going to be very difficult for you to control your acid levels in the body and this could mean that following the diet may not benefit you in the way you want, no matter how many alkalizing foods you consume. If you are going through too much stress, the best thing to do would be to consult a doctor and bring your stress levels in control before you start the diet plan.

To get the best out of your alkaline diet, it's important that you learn how to identify acidic food items and stay away from them. Apart from that, here are some basic tips you may want to follow in order to make the most out of the alkaline diet plan and lead a healthy life.

Eat Regularly
It is important for you to make time to eat regular and healthy meals if you want your body to get into control. No matter how busy you are, try to make time to ensure you eat the right amount of food multiple times a day rather than stuffing too much food two or three times a day.

Sleep Well
If you want to get healthy and want the alkaline diet to work, you need to provide your body with enough rest every day. You should try and get at least seven to eight hours of sleep because this helps relax your body and also relieves your body from a lot of acids, making you feel unhealthy.

Stop Smoking
If you want the alkaline diet to work, you need to say goodbye to your smoking habit so that it benefits you and you manage to make the diet a successful one. This will not only help you in weight loss but will also drive away diseases and increase your energy levels.

Low Levels of Nutrients in Foods Due to Industrial Farming
When you start to follow an alkaline diet, the one thing you may want to focus on is purchasing products that are organic and homegrown. Products that are available on an industrial level do not contain the

number of nutrients as you would want them to because they are mass produced and usually chemical based. Thankfully, there are farmer markets that are available in every locality and if there is one close to you, make the most of it and purchase all fresh fruits and vegetables from a farmer market so that you get homegrown and organic food products.

Low Levels of Fiber in the Diet
When you follow an alkaline diet, the one thing you need to make sure is that you provide your body with enough fiber so that it functions effectively and you manage to eliminate the dirty toxins that you are suffering from. If you want to lose weight during the alkaline diet, fiber plays an essential role in easing better digestion. Broccoli, apples, and carrots are high in fiber so when you start your diet, make sure to include plenty of these on a daily basis.

Including Non Grass-Fed Animal Meats in the Diet
It is not easy for a non-vegetarian to switch to an alkaline diet that is completely vegan and this is why you may want to cut down the amount of meat you include in your daily life without completely eliminating it. However, there are meat that are non grass-fed that you may want to try and avoid because these are higher in fat and calories. Grass-fed meat manages to provide you with proteins which benefit you. While your goal should be to give up on meat completely, you can always start by reducing the amount of meat you eat and choosing a flexitarian diet for a few days.

Eliminating Unnecessary Hormones from Your Life
In order for you to stay healthy, it is important to identify your exposure to hidden hormones. These hormones could be found in a variety of food items and beauty products as well as plastics that you are often exposed to. The best way to understand where the hidden hormones lie is to check for the level of chemicals in the product because that's what usually relates to as a hidden hormone. If you

want to lower the risk of exposure to these hidden hormones, you might want to try opting in for natural products, whether it's for food or your beauty products or even plastic and try to limit the amount of chemicals in your life.

Radiation
Electromagnetic radiation can cause a number of side effects in your life and while we believe we keep ourselves away from this exposure, the truth is there are a number of products you use on a daily basis including your cell phone and your microwave that release this radiation more than you would like them to. If you want to stay healthy, you should try to stop heating food in a microwave and make smaller portions that you finish up in one consumption. You should also sleep away from your cell phone so that it does not affect you while you sleep.

Preservatives in Food Coloring
While natural food coloring is still manageable, artificial food colors are full of chemicals and preservatives which do not work well on your body and may slow down the process of digestion. This also affects your vital organs which is why you should stay away from any product that has preservatives or artificial food coloring.

Pesticides
Pesticides are harmful to the environment and while a lot of people know this, what they don't realize is these pesticides can also be extremely harmful to the human body as well. Prolonged exposure to pesticides can lead to various health-related issues and can increase the risk of cancer. If you believe organic is something that is just a little more expensive, then you may want to reconsider because too much of pesticides could increase neurological disorders such as Parkinson's disease, leukemia, asthma, and other diseases in your body. An alkaline diet always recommends raw, organic and natural

foods as a force to the ones that are treated with pesticides for the obvious reasons.

Over-Exercise
It's common for people to feel pumped once they start any diet plan and they always like to accompany it with an exercise regime. While exercise is great, it's important for you to make sure you don't overdo it because an excess of anything will be bad and that is also true for exercise. If you attempt exercising more than your body can handle, you could end up with a muscle tear or tissue damage that could take months to heal. Instead of doing too much on one day, you may want to start slow but make sure that you don't miss a single day of exercise so that your body gets movement regularly and you manage to burn fat and increase your energy levels effectively.

Pollution
Although it is hard to stay away from pollution, this is something that could affect your body in various ways on a regular basis. High pollution levels can cause damage to your lungs, brain, and heart. The reason why an alkaline diet is recommended is because this helps clean your organs and increases the strength of your lungs as well as cleanses your heart and removes all the dirty toxins and pollutants from your body regularly.

Poor Chewing and Eating Habits
One of the worst things that you can do is to eat your food too quickly. The faster you swallow, the higher the chances of you staying overweight because it takes a while for bigger food particles to digest in the body as compared to smaller particles that you chew properly. It is also said that you should eat your food slower because this gives your body enough time to digest the food more effectively and drinking water in between your meals definitely helps you to stay fitter in comparison to those who start chewing and swallowing the food really fast.

Shallow Breathing

Most people lead a hectic life and they literally have no time to take a deep breath! If you want to stay healthy, it's important to breathe easily and with comfort rather than taking short breaths and trying to take in as much air in a short shallow breath as possible. The deeper your breaths are, the more relaxed your body is and the better it is for your lungs. In case you have a breathing problem and you are used to taking shorter breaths, you may want to start practicing taking deep breaths at least five to six times a day until you get into the habit of it.

With so many diet plans being introduced into the market on a regular basis, it is natural to get confused with regards to which one will work, and which ones make absolutely no sense! If you are looking to lose weight without staying concerned about your health, then you should probably look for something that works fast and has no logic to it. While these kinds of diet plan often attract more customers, they are the kind of diet plans that eventually fail because they don't live up to their expectations and once somebody gives up the diet, they get back to the way they were or even heavier.

The reason an alkaline diet is so perfectly crafted is because it doesn't just focus on losing weight, but it also includes crucial steps that help reduce and reverse the risks of life-threatening diseases including cancer and diabetes. An alkaline diet is the only diet that can help cure you from within and you will feel better and more energetic in no time.

An alkaline diet may be difficult to start off with but once you start it, you will realize how amazing you feel, and you'll never want to get off this diet plan in your life. One small step towards a healthy future can pave the path for a happy, stress-free, younger, energetic and beautiful you! Take that step today and adapt to an alkaline way of life!

Chapter 4 – Week One: Meal Plan and Recipes

Breakfast

Smoothies are the best way to really cleanse your body. They break down all of the ingredients so that your body can properly digest them, getting as many vitamins, minerals, and other nutrients as possible.

Use Ziploc bags or other containers to prep this recipe. You can buy your ingredients in bulk, portion them out, and keep them stowed away for when you are ready. You can alternate types of smoothies as well so that you can have something a little different every morning.

Rather than using mixed berries, you can also pick one type of berry to stick to for this recipe. Mixed berries often come in freezer bags, giving you some blend rich in antioxidants. These will usually contain raspberries, blackberries, blueberries, and strawberries. Buying all of these fresh can be challenging so, if you do not want a frozen blend, you can stick to simply one or two kinds of berries.

Both the spinach and the berries in this will be very detoxifying. These are packed with antioxidants that help to reduce inflammation. In addition, the spinach isn't going to add that much of a flavor. The coconut oil can help to make it smooth and there are many health benefits to this type of healthy fat as well.

The chia seeds and the green tea are going to help you kick start your weight loss while also keeping you full until lunch. These are very simple ingredients that can be added to many different recipes in order to help you fight off cravings. Chia seeds are also great for your skin and hair. They add a great texture and an almost sweet taste.

Detoxing Berry Smoothie

Ingredients
- 1 cup chopped spinach
- 1 cup green tea (brewed and chilled)
- 1 avocado
- 1 cup mixed berries
- 1 tablespoon freshly chopped mint (optional)
- 1 teaspoon coconut oil
- 1 tablespoon chia seeds

Directions
1. Pour ingredients into a blender and pulse until smooth. Blend with ice if it is not cold enough at the time you make it.

2. Make a double serving and have it ready for the next day. You can also make it in batches and freeze it or you can prep the ingredients in containers and blend them fresh every morning.

Lunch

This recipe is really going to help clean you out. It gives you the energy needed to make it through the day, vitamins, and minerals to rebalance the good nutrients in your body and tastes great on top of all that! The soupiness of this recipe will help ensure that you are kept cleaned out with a fast-working digestive system.

If you are sick, this is a great one. It will replenish your body with what is needed to fight off all the toxins that might exist within your immune system.

The spinach is here again, but this time, cooked down. You will notice how cooking the spinach really brings out a new flavor. It doesn't have a slimy texture either, even though it is cooked in the soup. The cabbage has a really strong flavor as well.

This soup will help you see that all these green ingredients can still make something exceptionally tasty. Sprinkle with vegan cheese or pair with toasted whole-wheat bread if you want to spice up the meal even more!

Cabbage Cleansing Soup
Ingredients
- ½ head of cabbage
- ½ large white onion
- 4 cloves garlic
- 3 large carrots
- 1 cup chopped parsley
- 1 cup chopped spinach
- 6 cups water and 1 vegetable bouillon cube
- Or 6 cups vegetable stock
- 1 teaspoon Paprika
- 1 teaspoon Red pepper flakes
- Salt/pepper to taste
- 1 tablespoon oil

Directions
1. Start by mincing your garlic and onion. Dump this into a large pot with your oil and start to cook on medium heat. Add oil as needed to ensure they do not burn or stick.
2. While that is cooking, you can chop the rest of your veggies. Your cabbage should be shredded, though cutting it into cubes is fine as well. Simply ensure that the pieces will be small enough for a spoon.

3. For chopping the carrots, either do bite-sized cubes or thick slices.

4. Chop the parsley and spinach finely as well.

5. Once the onions have started to become transparent and fragrant, add the water and bouillon cube, or the vegetable stock.

6. Add the rest of your ingredients as well.

7. Allow this to cook on high heat for an hour, stirring frequently, or medium for two hours, stirring less frequently.

8. Add salt, pepper, and more red pepper flakes to taste.

9. This will be good for five days in the refrigerator. After cooling, ensure that you only reheat one serving at a time.

Dinner

A zoodle machine will be your best friend as you go on your weight loss journey. Food like spaghetti, Fettuccini Alfredo, macaroni and cheese, and other pasta can be hard to resist. These are usually high in carbohydrates, however, especially if you are eating white pasta. Whole wheat pasta is great for you as well but using vegetable noodles is a way to ensure even fewer carbs and calories are consumed on your weight loss diet.

This recipe is going to be refreshing and calming for a nice nightly dinner. The lemon will make you feel reinvigorated, and the zoodles help to keep you hydrated. Once you learn how to make zoodles, you won't even want to go back to the way it was before!

You can also eat it cold the next day if you would like! This can be a great lunch if you are looking to switch things up. You could swap it with the soup for a night as well!

The key here is going to be the fresh herbs, garlic, and lemon. The zoodles won't have much of a flavor on their own; instead, it will be the texture that's important. The other ingredients will really help to give it a flavor that stands out night after night of eating.

Add a vegan cheese substitute as well. Experiment with different toppings you could add that would really help to spice this up.

Fresh Lemon Zoodles

Ingredients
- 1-pound zucchini
- ½ pound cherry tomatoes
- 5 garlic cloves
- 1 lemon
- ½ cup chopped parsley

- 1 tablespoon oil
- Salt and pepper to taste

Directions

1. Start by preparing your zoodles. This will be done with a zoodle maker. If you do not have one, do not worry. You can simply peel your zucchini and then cut it into strips. You can also use a peeler to shave it down and use these strips for your noodles.

2. Pour the oil into your pan. Toss in the zoodles and minced garlic.

3. Squeeze half of the lemon into the pan. Ensure the zoodles do not become too brown or else they won't reheat right.

4. Allow these to cook till they turn light brown.

5. While these are cooking, slice your cherry tomatoes in half.

6. Serve while warm, topped with cherry tomatoes and fresh parsley.

7. Squeeze the other half of the lemon over the dish and use salt and pepper to taste.

8. These will be good for four days in the fridge.

Grocery List

- 2 bunches spinach or 1 bag
- 1 avocado
- About ½ pound mixed berries
- Fresh bunch of each: mint, parsley,
- ½ head of cabbage, or 1 bag chopped cabbage

- ½ large white onion
- 1 bulb garlic
- 3 large carrots
- 1-pound zucchini
- ½ pound cherry tomatoes
- 1 lemon

Chapter 5 – Week Two: Reactivate

You will start to see that as you simplify your recipes, your pallet becomes more sensitive to the great flavors of garlic, onion, pepper, and more. When we are eating processed or other junk foods, it can mess up our pallet because these foods are often loaded with salt and sugar.

This week is going to be focused on bringing out some of your body's natural weight loss processes. These foods are going to be rich in nutrients and most importantly, filled with ingredients that keep you full for longer.

As you start to eat healthier you will notice that it becomes easier to stay focused as well. This is because you aren't as hungry, and your cravings will begin to subside. You might realize that you can get work done more efficiently or that you are more likely to exercise because you are able to focus a lot easier. The better you eat, the better you are going to feel!

Breakfast

This is one that you are going to want to prep overnight. I find that overnight breakfasts work best for me because I am taking care of my future self. When you wake up in the morning, knowing that there is a delicious breakfast waiting for you will make it that much easier to get out of bed.

This pudding is great because it is loaded with chia seeds. These are going to keep you feeling full throughout the day so you won't be tempted to snack a ton before lunch.

What I love about this pudding is that it is also super easy to customize. You can keep it healthy and add whichever fruit toppings you might like. Perhaps you make it themed like strawberry banana or cranberry apple.

You could even add raspberries to this one to make it sort of a raspberry lemonade flavor. Not only is this a good breakfast but it can be a dessert as well! Add peanut butter, Nutella, or something else indulgent when you want a sweet snack. Whatever you choose, it is totally up to you!

Lemon Chia Detox Pudding

Ingredients
- 1/2 cup chia seeds
- 2 cups non-dairy milk
- ½ tablespoon sweetener of your choice
- 1 teaspoon vanilla extract
- 2 tablespoons lemon juice

Directions
1. Mix everything together at once and put it in an airtight container. Let this sit for about ten minutes.

2. After this, stir it well and reseal. Place in the fridge for at least three hours but overnight is a good idea so you can have it for breakfast.

3. Experiment with different toppings!

Lunch

Kale can be something that new plant-based eaters are turned off by. It doesn't have the most appealing name, and without seasoning or dressing, it can be a bit plain. However, it is packed with nutrients and has a salty taste that can be satisfying when combined with the right flavors.

Double up on the dressing for this and make an entire bottle you can keep in the fridge! It is the easiest dressing to make for salad and one that is a lifesaver on days when I don't have anything in the fridge but some extra lettuce and other veggies.

Like most recipes in this book, you can customize this one more to your liking as well. Kale is a really salty vegetable when used right so pair it with sweet veggies like red peppers to give your pallet a completely balanced taste.

Clean Kale Salad

Ingredients
- About 7 cups chopped kale (10 ounces)
- ½ red onion
- 2 large carrots
- 1 red pepper
- ½ cup chopped cilantro
- ¼ cup chopped almonds
- 1 lemon
- 3 minced garlic cloves
- 2 tablespoons oil
- Salt and pepper to taste

Directions
1. Start by chopping your kale if you purchased it in bunches.

2. Dice your onion and carrots as well. Save half the onion for dinner.

3. Cube your red pepper.

4. Chop the cilantro and almonds finely as well.

5. Now it is time to assemble your salad or meal prep containers. Start with the kale, then add carrots, pepper, cilantro, and onions. Place a paper towel on top if you want to keep them dry.

6. Keep the onions in a separate container.

7. Now it is time to make the dressing. Mix together the juice from 1 squeezed lemon, the oil, and the minced garlic cloves. This dressing will be best if it can sit for a night so the oil and lemon absorb the flavors of the garlic.

8. Wait to pour your dressing on your salad till right before you eat to ensure your kale stays crisp!

Dinner

To make sure I'm eating healthy, I like to have a rainbow on my plate when I eat. The more colorful something is, the healthier I know it will be. However, green is going to be your most important color. An all green plate isn't an all bad thing, remember that. That said, it can get a little boring when that's the only thing you are eating.

That's why I love this rainbow cauliflower rice bowl. It also has a great dressing which you could make extra of to keep a bottle on hand as well. What is great about the plant-based movement is that more stores are coming out with products to cater to your needs. This includes pre-packaged cauliflower rice, which can be found in many freezer sections.

Rice is good but only when it is wild or brown blended. All white rice can be over-filling and starchy and doesn't offer you as many health benefits. Cauliflower rice is an even healthier choice. It has a great texture with little flavor, helping you use the veggies and sauces you choose in your stir-fry as a way to satisfy your cravings.

If you want this for an entire week, double up the veggies and save half before cooking. You will then be able to simply toss them with oil and sauce after they have been frozen.

Rainbow Cauliflower Rice Bowl

Ingredients
- 1 head cauliflower
- 5 cloves garlic
- 1 red pepper
- 2 large carrots
- 1 yellow squash
- ½ cup chopped cilantro.
- ½ red onion

- 6 teaspoons soy sauce
- 6 teaspoons water
- 2 tablespoons sweetener
- 2 teaspoons hot sauce
- 1 teaspoon sesame oil
- 1 tablespoon oil of your choice

Directions
1. Start by grinding your cauliflower rice down with a shredder or crumble it yourself. Some locations will also have cauliflower already turned into rice for you.

2. Mince the garlic and dice the onion. Pour all these into a pan on medium heat with the tablespoon of oil of your choice.

3. Chop the pepper, carrots, and squash. Cube these into bite-size pieces.

4. Add the cauliflower rice to the pan, along with more oil to ensure these stay coated as well.

5. Once the "rice" starts to become brown, add the rest of the vegetables. Add water as it needs more moisture, but not too much, because as the squash and carrots cook they will release more moisture as well. Add salt and pepper to taste, sampling a veggie to get the right amount.

6. Cook these for a while as you start making the dressing. Mix together the soy sauce, water, sweetener, hot sauce, and sesame oil.

7. Pull the veggies off the stove when they have been thoroughly cooked. Portion out your meal so that you have three servings left.

8. Top with dressing and cilantro. This will be good for the next four days.

Grocery List
- 2 lemons
- About 7 cups chopped kale (10 ounces)

- 1 red onion
- 4 large carrots
- 1 red pepper
- 1 bunch each: cilantro
- 1 garlic bulb
- 1 head cauliflower
- 5 cloves garlic
- 1 yellow squash

Chapter 6 - Week Three: Rebuild

This is going to be an antioxidant, vitamin C heavy week. We are going to build your immune system so that it can help keep your body regulated and healthy. When you can ensure all of your systems are taken care of, then you do not have to worry about underlying issues delaying your weight loss.

Sometimes, we might think we're eating healthy when in reality our food choices are causing us to keep the weight on for longer. If you are not choosing the right healthy foods, then there's no point in doing it in the first place! These plant-based recipes are based on whole foods that are going to keep you filled with nutrients and energized enough to make it through your day.

Breakfast

This smoothie is another great way to help clean you out while also awakening your inner systems. The orange is powerful because it is loaded with Vitamin C. Oranges are incredibly sweet as well so you might not even want to add any sweetener.

Oranges are also great to include in your diet on their own as snacks. This recipe calls for two oranges and they will give you two servings when making this drink. You can buy extra and keep them around for the aforementioned snack as well. They will help keep you hydrated and vitamin C has actually been proven to help you lose weight even faster because fat burns at a higher rate when vitamin C levels are normal.

In the last chapter, we discussed how it is important to make sure that your plate is colorful, like a rainbow, in order to provide you with all the proper nutrients. Since everything is blended together, it is easier to not worry about color variety here.

Instead, when building a smoothie, it can be helpful to focus on including colors that are all the same. This way, you can see how they will be able to better complement each other. Ginger is great to add because it has so many healing properties. It can help you feel better in general while also ensuring that you are reducing inflammation and any feelings of nausea you might experience in the morning.

Powerful Ginger Turmeric Smoothie

Ingredients

- 2 oranges
- 1 teaspoon ginger
- 1 teaspoon turmeric
- 1 carrot
- 1 tablespoon chia seeds
- 2 teaspoons sweetener (optional)
- 1 cup ice

Directions

1. Peel your oranges and break them apart so that they blend a bit easier.

2. Blend these with the ice and chia seeds.

3. Once you do not see any large chunks of orange left, add the remainder of the ingredients and blend.

4. Drink half and save the rest for the next day. Double or triple the recipe and freeze it for faster mornings.

Lunch

Once again, we're going to focus on a very color-oriented dish. This is great because it is filled with tomatoes, which can actually help reduce your appetite. Soup isn't always filling enough for everyone but this one will certainly satisfy your needs.

The high acidity of the tomatoes and peppers will also help to reduce your overall levels of bloating. This can make you look physically slimmer, so after this week, there's a chance you will start to see some of the physical effects of your kick-started weight loss.

Not only that but the tomatoes and peppers are sweet, giving this a great flavor. Both of these vegetables are great on their own because they provide so many flavor-packed bites. Combining them gives you a unique experience and the added garlic and herbs will help make this an even better treat. If you aren't fully vegan, it wouldn't hurt to have a grilled cheese with this or you can substitute a non-dairy cheese as well.

Top this delicious soup with croutons for a crunch and remember that crackers can always go great with soup. Try making this again with green or yellow roasted peppers to see if there is a big difference in flavor.

Rebuilding Red Soup

Ingredients
- 2 red peppers
- 2 cans low sodium diced tomatoes
- 1 small white onion
- 6 cloves garlic
- 2 cups water and veggie bouillon cube or 2 cups veggie stock
- Red pepper flakes to taste
- 3 teaspoons paprika

- Salt and pepper to taste

Directions
1. Start by roasting your red peppers. Chop them into quarters and massage them with oil. Put them in the oven at 400 degrees for about 15 minutes. When the skins start to shrivel you will know they're done.

2. Now, start to cook your onion and garlic, minced, with just a dash of oil to keep them from burning in the pot.

3. While these are cooking, peel the skins off your red peppers and toss them with the tomatoes in a food processor.

4. Add this mixture, with the water/veggie stock and paprika to the pot with the onions.

5. Cook on high heat for an hour, or medium heat for two hours. Continually stir and add red pepper flakes, as well as salt and pepper, to taste. The redder the pepper flakes, the spicier the soup will be.

6. This will stay good for four days when refrigerated but you can freeze to keep it lasting longer.

Dinner

Taco night is a big deal in many people's homes for a reason. While tacos aren't always the best for weight loss, this enchilada casserole can be the next best thing. This recipe can be great with many different kinds of toppings.

You could pair it with chips and salsa or use guacamole as a dip/topping as well. Whatever you might choose is completely up to you. This is a great recipe for those individuals that are hesitant to try a plant-based diet. You might introduce it to friends and show them that they can eat healthily, focused on plants, just as well.

Loaded Enchilada Casserole

Ingredients
- 1 white onion
- 6 cloves garlic
- 1 can corn
- 1 can black beans
- 1 green pepper
- ½ jalapeño
- 2 large heirloom tomatoes
- 4 small cans tomato sauce
- ½ tablespoon each: chili pepper, cumin, garlic powder
- 10 whole-wheat or corn tortillas of your choice
- 1 cup vegan cheese

Directions
1. Ensure that the oven has been preheated to 350 degrees Fahrenheit.

2. Use a regular rectangle baking dish and line with foil or nonstick spray as needed.
3. Use a medium pan to cook the diced onion and garlic. Use about a tablespoon of oil or water/broth of your choice.

4. Chop the pepper, jalapeño, and tomatoes. They should be diced and mixed together along with the corn and black beans. Ensure the corn and black beans have been drained and rinsed.

5. Add this mixture to the garlic and onions, cooking it all so that the peppers become soft.

6. In a separate bowl, mix together the tomato sauce and seasoning. This is going to be your sauce so taste it to make sure that it isn't too spicy but is still spicy enough.

7. Now it will be time to assemble your casserole. Start by coating the dish in tomato sauce. Add a layer of tortillas and then a layer of the veggie mixture. The first layer will probably take about 6 tortillas. Make sure it covers the bottom and the sides as well. It doesn't have to be perfect but ensure it is covered enough to hold the rest of the veggie mix. Cut it into strips if it makes it easier for you to cover the dish.

8. Add a second layer of tortillas, about four, to cover the veggie mix. Add the remaining mix, and top with vegan cheese of your choice.

9. Bake for about twenty minutes or until the cheese is brown.

10. Serve right away and freeze the rest if you can't finish it within four days.

Grocery List
- 2 oranges
- 1 teaspoon ginger
- 1 teaspoon turmeric
- 1 carrot
- 2 red peppers
- 2 cans low sodium diced tomatoes
- 2 small white onions
- 1 bulb garlic
- 1 can corn
- 1 can black beans

- 1 green pepper
- ½ jalapeño
- 2 large heirloom tomatoes
- 4 small cans tomato sauce
- 10 whole-wheat or corn tortillas of your choice
- 1 cup vegan cheese of your choice

Chapter 7 – Week Four: Rebalance

This week will be focused on helping you transition back into normal everyday eating after having eaten lighter for the past three weeks. What you have to remember about losing weight is that it shouldn't always be temporary. If you are looking to lose fifteen or so pounds, you might stick to a shorter diet. However, if you are overweight, want to lose a lot of weight, and want to keep the weight off, it is all about changing your lifestyle.

In the first three weeks, you were eating things that were completely clean and focused on whole veggies that helped to burn fat. Now, we're going to give you recipes that are made with foods you might have eaten before your plant-based diet, only this time around, a lot healthier. This can help to ensure that you are remaining focused on your diet while also eating the fun things you would if you weren't trying to lose weight.

This food will still help you lose weight, but now you are going to balance it back with food that you would want to eat every day. The more you can find alternates to the things you used to eat, the easier it will be to actually stick to a healthier lifestyle.

Breakfast

Cereal is a huge craving for many people. The problem with store-bought cereal is that it is loaded with sugar. It shouldn't even be considered breakfast at certain points because it contains so much added sugar and other food dyes, especially in cereals aimed at kids.

If you choose healthier store-bought cereal, this can sometimes end up being plain, or it might include other additives that make it unhealthy for reasons not just including the amount of added sugar.

This cereal is one that you can keep around in your pantry for a long time. You can simply eat it plain as a breakfast or a snack. It also pairs nicely with a whole fruit on the side.

Chop up fruit to add on top as well. Strawberries and bananas always go great in cereal because they do well with the cold milk. It is even great without milk and simply eaten as a snack.

Simple Crispy Flaked Cereal

Ingredients
- 2 cups whole wheat flour, or flour of your choice
- 2 cups wheat bran
- 3 tablespoons chia seeds
- 1 teaspoon baking powder
- Dash of salt
- 1/3 cup sweetener of your choice
- ½ cup non-dairy milk of your choice

Directions
1. Start by making sure that the oven has been preheated to 350 degrees Fahrenheit.

2. In a large mixing bowl, combine the dry ingredients which include the flour, bran, seeds, powder, and dash of salt.

3. Once this has been mixed, add your sweetener, milk, and about a cup of water as well, more or less depending on the consistency.

4. The consistency should be like a dough, such as cookie dough. Anything too wet isn't going to bake right.

5. This is a lot of cereal, so you can freeze half for the next week.

6. The other half roll as flat as possible onto your baking sheet. You can press it down with a spoon or you could put wax paper over the top to make sure it doesn't get stuck to the rolling pin.

7. It should be about as thin as cereal flakes would be.

8. Bake these for about fifteen minutes, pull them out if they start to look brown.

9. Let these cool. Once cooled, cut them into cubes so that they are the shape that cereal would be.

10. Now, you will want to bake them again at a reduced 300 degrees. Cook for about 5 minutes at a time, stirring them in between.

11. After about fifteen minutes they should be crispy.

12. Let cool and serve with milk. They'll be good for about a week, though they might get soggy.

Lunch

As we've already discussed, berries can hold some great anti-inflammatory properties. This is perfect for anyone that is looking to lose weight because it decreases bloating. There are many other healing properties to foods loaded with antioxidants besides simply losing weight as well, such as their benefit to your immune system.

What I love about blueberries and blackberries is that they don't always need to be used in sweet things. They might be super sweet when added with sugar but paired with other savory things, they can add an interesting twist.

Apple cider vinegar is another food that has great properties. It will give your dishes the flavor needed to counteract any other blandness that might be present. It helps to preserve your food a bit as well, so salads like these will last a little longer in the fridge when tossed with ACV.

Anti-Inflammatory Berry Salad

Ingredients
- 1 cup blueberries
- 1 cup blackberries
- 1 can black-eyed peas
- 1 can corn
- 1 cup chopped cilantro
- 1 red onion
- 1 can red kidney beans
- 4 tablespoons oil
- 2 tablespoons apple cider vinegar
- 1 teaspoon sweetener
- Salt and pepper to taste

Directions

1. Ensure all of the canned food has been drained and rinsed. This includes the peas, beans, and corn.

2. Chop the cilantro and onion.

3. Chop any especially large berries, but they should be the right size.

4. Mix the berries, peas, corn, cilantro, onion, and beans in a bowl.

5. Toss with the vinegar, oil, and sweetener.
6. Add salt and pepper to taste. Add red pepper flakes if you want an extra kick as well.

Dinner

Chili seems like such a comfort food, especially when you picture loading it with cheese, crackers, sour cream, and other decadent toppings. While all this is nice, you do not have to do all that just to have a delicious chili.

This is one that is filled with flavors to keep your pallet interested. You can still add any of the above mentioned but look for vegan substitutes so that you can better stick to your diet.

This is going to be loaded with foods to help keep your system regulated while also kick starting your weight loss goals. Freeze it in portioned containers, because it reheats really well. It is a great meal to always have as a backup when you need something simple and quick, too.

Power Chili

Ingredients

- 1 onion
- 6 cloves garlic
- 1 can black beans
- 1 can corn
- 1 can diced tomatoes
- 1 small can tomato sauce
- ½ jalapeño
- 1/2 cup veggie stock
- 1 tablespoon oil
- 1 package tofu, regular
- ½ tablespoon each: cumin, chili powder, paprika

Directions

1. The first thing you are going to do is cook your tofu. You can do this in a skillet if you want to cook the chili in a slow cooker or you can cook it directly in the pot that you will add the rest of your ingredients to.

2. Crumble it with a wooden spoon so it is the consistency that ground beef might be.

3. Dice the garlic and onion, as well as the jalapeño.

4. Cook this with the oil, veggie stock, cumin, chili powder, paprika, and garlic and onion.

5. Cook the mix until it is brown and then add together with black beans, corn, tomatoes, and jalapeño.

6. Pour the tomato sauce over the mixture and cook for at least an hour.

7. Eat as soon as it is warm and keep in the fridge for about four days.

8. Freeze it and heat later as well!

Grocery List
- 2 cups wheat bran
- 2 cups whole wheat flour, or flour of your choice (if not already in pantry)
- 1 cup blueberries
- 1 cup blackberries
- 1 can black-eyed peas
- 2 cans corn
- 1 bunch chopped cilantro
- 1 red onion

- 1 white onion
- 1 can red kidney beans
- 2 tablespoons apple cider vinegar
- 6 cloves garlic
- 1 can black beans
- 1 can diced tomatoes
- 1 small can tomato sauce
- 1 jalapeño
- 1 package tofu, regular

Chapter 8 - Week Five – Relax

Congratulations! You did it! You completed a four-week program to help kick start both your weight loss and your plant-based diet. By now, you have reset your body so that it is more balanced in nutrients and hormones. This is going to make it all the easier to continue to lose the weight and keep it off.

Do not get discouraged if you find that you aren't losing as much weight now as you were in the beginning. A lot of the weight loss in the beginning was water weight, so you won't lose it as fast throughout the rest of your journey.

That doesn't mean you have to stop on the path to reducing your weight even further, either. Instead, you can find comforting, decadent, and indulgent food that is still going to help you reduce your weight! This chapter is all about celebrating your weight loss without worrying about falling back into bad habits.

This food is a little simpler, meaning it won't be packed with as much of the good stuff. However, it is still going to be plant-based, meaning that it will help in reducing weight overall.

Breakfast

Overnight oats are a great way to experiment with different types of flavors. Just like the chia pudding, this is perfect for the morning. All you have to do is mix some ingredients together and throw it in the fridge! It is an on-the-go breakfast as well if you want to simply toss it in your bag and eat it at work.

I used to think I didn't like oatmeal but that was because I was using instant oatmeal. When you use the method of creating overnight oats, it is going to help bring out more flavors and have a smoother texture. It is also a bigger serving and these healthy oats are going to ensure that you are feeling fuller all day.

You can make them with fruits and dried toppings, like crystallized ginger or coconut flakes. You could also make them more indulgent, like a dessert, with chocolate chips or caramel cinnamon drizzle. Whatever you choose to do, enjoy these tasty overnight oats!

Coconut Carrots Overnight Oats

Ingredients
- 1 cup oats – rolled
- One carrot
- ½ cups dried coconut
- 1 tablespoon sweetener of your choice
- 1 ½ cup non-dairy milk
- ½ teaspoon ginger
- ½ teaspoon vanilla
- 2 teaspoons cinnamon

Directions
1. This is something that you are going to want to get started the night before. All you have to do is get an airtight container and fill it with all of the ingredients, except the carrot and coconut flakes.

2. Mix the ingredients well. Smell to test if you need to add more cinnamon or ginger.

3. Enjoy the next morning heated up or cold! Add the coconut flakes and shred the carrot on top along with any extra seasoning or sweetener to get it to your liking.

Lunch

Avocado toast is filling, easy, and versatile. Whenever you are in doubt of what to make for lunch, this can be a great option. Avocados are full of healthy fat that keeps your body consistently losing weight. They are plain enough to customize, but the texture and the flavor that is there still keeps this dish interesting.

You can experiment by using this as a breakfast, too. Add an egg if you are not completely plant-based. You can also use avocado toast as a side dish. This recipe will call for two slices but you can simply use one and save half the avocado for a later date. You might also find that you do not want an entire avocado either and use half to spread between the two different slices of toast.

You could even make it dinner if you want to add a protein source. This could quickly turn into a sandwich with the right sauces and proteins. For now, we are going to focus on an easy and quick recipe that will surprise your taste buds.

Rich Radish Avocado Toast

Ingredients
- 1 avocado
- 2 slices of whole wheat toast
- 2 radishes
- ½ cup sprouts
- Italian seasoning
- Balsamic vinaigrette (to taste)

Directions
1. Toast your bread to your desired level.

2. Cut the avocado in half, putting a slice on each side.

3. Mash your avocado into the toast with a fork.

4. Slice your radishes thin and layer them in two rows across the toast. One radish should cover each slice.

5. Add sprouts and season with Italian seasoning, as well as salt and pepper to taste.

6. Drizzle with balsamic vinaigrette.

7. This can't be saved as the avocado will brown, but it is very easy to assemble every morning.

Dinner

What better way to celebrate your success than with a creamy and decadent Alfredo sauce? There are seemingly very few health benefits to traditional Alfredo, as it is a heavy cream and cheese-based sauce. However, when you make this dish, you will realize that you do not need cheese to have a tasty Alfredo.

The spaghetti squash can be too minimal for some but that is where the cashews come in. These are high in protein and are going to combat the lack of filling carbs from the spaghetti squash.

On top of that, you will also find that the fiber from the broccoli works to keep you fuller for longer. Experiment with what you decide to add to your Alfredo dishes as well. Roasted red pepper or even roasted instead of cooked garlic can be enough to really switch this up.

You might also experiment by adding different plant-based proteins, such as tempeh or tofu. You could try a buffalo Alfredo by adding hot sauce or even pair it with barbequed veggies for a summer twist. Do not be afraid of the possibilities that come along with this easy sauce!

Best Broccoli Alfredo Spaghetti Squash

Ingredients

- 1 spaghetti squash
- 2 cups broccoli
- 1 cup cashews
- 6 garlic cloves
- ½ onion
- 3 tablespoons yeast
- ¼ cup non-dairy milk

- 2 tablespoons Italian seasoning

Directions

1. At least six hours before you plan to make this, start soaking your cashews in about a cup of water. Alternately, you can begin soaking them the night before.

2. Start by preheating the oven to 400 degrees. This is for cooking your spaghetti squash.

3. Now, cut your spaghetti squash in half. Usually, one half is a good serving so the other can be saved for tomorrow or you can cook it all at once now.

4. Scoop out the insides, including the seeds.

5. Rub down the inside with olive oil and add a dash of salt and pepper as well.

6. Lay it flat on a baking sheet and roast for about thirty minutes.

7. While this is cooking, you can start to cook the broccoli as well. First, chop any large pieces of broccoli and dice the onions and garlic, leaving two garlic cloves whole and setting them aside.

8. Add these all to a pan, along with a little oil to keep them from sticking.

9. As both the broccoli and squash are cooking, add the soaked cashews (after draining excess water), yeast, 2 whole garlic cloves, Italian seasoning, and non-dairy milk to a food processor or blender. Blend until smooth and creamy.

10. Add this to the broccoli and onions and cook on low as the spaghetti squash finishes up.

11. Once the spaghetti squash is done, pull it out and shred it with your fork so that it looks like thin noodles.

12. Add a spoonful of the sauce to each half and mix well with your fork.

13. Set half the sauce aside for later. There are about four servings of the sauce for this recipe.

14. Distribute the remaining half between both spaghetti squash halves.

15. If you prefer, you can add any non-dairy cheese at this point.

16. Bake again for about 10 minutes, or until the top starts to brown.

17. Enjoy!

18. You can make all four spaghetti squash servings at once and they will still be good to eat, but they will taste better served fresh.

Grocery List
- 1 cup oats – rolled
- One carrot
- ½ cup dried coconut
- 1 avocado per day of having avocado toast
- 1 loaf of bread- whole wheat
- 1 bunch radishes
- ½ pound sprouts

- Balsamic vinaigrette of your choice
- 1 spaghetti squash per 2 days of meal plan
- 1 head broccoli per day of meal plan
- 1 bulb of garlic (only 6 cloves needed if you have some from last week)
- 1 small onion

Chapter 9 - Bonus Recipes – Snacks and Treats

The reason some people struggle to lose weight isn't always because of the meals but because of the snacks that they eat in between. It can become really easy to lose track of the things that we are eating and sneaky calories might pop into your diet through candy, chips, and sodas. These snack recipes are going to keep you full and safe from your cravings so that you can focus on sticking to your diet.

Some will only need an extra few items aside what's already in your pantry as well. They might even be made from leftover ingredients that you had on your shopping list. They are all rather easy and though they might not be the healthiest option, they are better than starving yourself or choosing something entirely unhealthy instead.

Peanut Butter Banana Ice Cream

Even if it is a Saturday morning and you want ice cream for breakfast, you do not have to worry about breaking your diet. This ice cream only has three ingredients and can really taste like the real deal.

Ice cream can be so tempting, especially in the summer when you frequently see others licking their cones. Do not be afraid of ice cream anymore with this guilt-free version! It doesn't even include any sweetener, though you could certainly add some if you are looking for a more indulgent twist.

This ice cream is just as versatile as the ice cream you might buy in a store. You could use carob chips or a drizzle of chocolate syrup to make it extra sweet. You could include oats or cookie crumbs to give it a tasty crunch. Keep this around in your freezer so that you are never tempted to break your diet and eat other unhealthy sweets.

Ingredients
- 4 bananas, sliced and frozen
- 1 cup peanut butter
- 1 teaspoon vanilla

Directions
1. Start by slicing your bananas and freezing them. You could buy frozen bananas or you can do it yourself by using parchment paper and a baking sheet to freeze them.

2. Once frozen, blend the bananas, adding the peanut butter and vanilla half way through.

3. Freeze again for about an hour, mixing to see if it is the right consistency. Freeze for thirty-minute intervals until it is hard.

4. Enjoy within two weeks, if it manages to stay in your freezer for that long.

Sweet Potato Fries – 2 Ways

For this recipe, we are giving you two different ways that you can cook sweet potatoes as a snack. The first one is going to be by making fries. Fries can be one of the many things that break people's diets. They seem so harmless but all the added oil and salt can make all your other diet efforts fruitless. The second way is by making chips and another insidious side dish that could interrupt your diet unless you use a healthy recipe like this one.

You can make these "loaded" with chives or vegan cheese. You can add toppings like jalapenos to give them an extra kick. This goes for both the fries and the chips. These are perfect sides to black bean burgers or could be a meal on their own if you load them up with other important veggies.

You could even toss them with cinnamon and sugar in order to have a sweet snack. The best thing about sweet potatoes is that they are rather inexpensive as well. You can simply pick one up at the store and keep it on hand for whenever you are feeling attacked by a craving.

Ingredients
- 2 sweet potatoes
- 1 tablespoon oil
- Salt and pepper to taste

Directions for Fries:
1. Start by preheating the oven to 425 degrees.

2. Clean up your sweet potatoes with water, cutting out any big brown holes or bruises.

3. Peel and slice the sweet potatoes so that they are in the shape of fries.

4. Toss the fries with oil and seasoning.

5. Line a baking sheet with foil or use a nonstick spray to ensure the potatoes do not stick.

6. Place these on the sheet ensuring they aren't touching each other.

7. Bake for fifteen minutes. Flip then bake for fifteen more or until they've reached desired crispiness.

8. These will be good for three days and will serve about two to three snacks.

Directions for Chips

1. After cleaning the potatoes, slice them thinly so they are the thickness of potato chips.

2. Toss them with oil and seasoning again and line a baking sheet. Just like the fries, do not let them touch.

3. Bake for 10 minutes at 400 degrees. Flip them and bake for ten more minutes.

4. These will be good for about a week, though they might become soggy after four days or so.

Easy Pea Guacamole

When the idea of a pea guacamole first came about, some people were actually offended! How could you not include the creamy avocado in this decadent dish? Well, there is a way to avoid the hefty price tag that can sometimes come along with a good avocado.

There are times when they might be on sale yet they're too firm or too brown, making them hard to use anyway. What you can do is choose peas, which are relatively inexpensive. Use this with pita chips, tortilla chips, or any veggie when you want a snack or side dish.

Ingredients

- 2 cup peas
- 4 garlic cloves
- ½ cup chopped cilantro
- 1 jalapeño
- 2 tablespoons oil
- 2 tablespoons lime juice
- ½ teaspoon each: paprika, cumin, chili powder

Directions

1. First, chop your jalapeño, removing all seeds and inner meat.

2. Add all ingredients to a food processor and mix well.

3. Serve with chips or veggies of your choice.

Salty Edamame and Sauce

Edamame is a great snack to keep you full throughout the day. It is pretty easy to make, and many stores will even have frozen edamame. This means you can keep it around in your freezer for a long time to come so that you always have a snack on hand.

This is just one of many kinds of sauces that you could use with them as well. Do not be afraid to purchase new hot sauces and other dips for your edamame to ensure that you are always switching things up and keeping it interesting.

Ingredients
- 2 cups edamame
- ¼ cup soy sauce
- 1 tablespoon sweetener of your choice
- 2 teaspoons garlic powder
- ½ tablespoon salt

Directions
1. Whisk everything together except the edamame. Set aside.

2. Bring a pot of water to a boil, adding edamame and salt.

3. Once the edamame has become very green, usually after 4 minutes, remove and drain. Sprinkle with more salt.

4. Dip your edamame in the sauce, eating the beans out of the casing.

5. Only cook enough edamame the amount that you would like to eat, as it will not store well.

Pina Colada Popsicles

These are great for a party, or for yourself! They're non-alcoholic, but of course, you can customize them to not be if you want! These combine the great flavors of coconut and pineapple that Pina Colada lovers desire.

You will need popsicle molds, which can be great to have around. Popsicles can simply be made with coconut milk, sweetener, and the fruit of your choice. If you have these popsicle molds around, you can make these whenever you have an extra can of coconut milk or fruit that you need to use before it goes bad.

These popsicles are also great because they are pre-portioned out for you, meaning that you won't be as tempted to overeat.

Ingredients
- 1 cup pineapple
- 14 ounces coconut milk (full-fat)
- 2 tablespoons sweetener
- About 1 cup coconut flakes

Directions
1. For this, you will need molds and sticks for popsicles.

2. Start by chopping the pineapple into chunks.

3. Blend 1 cup pineapple with 14 ounces of coconut milk, usually around one can, along with 2 tablespoons of your sweetener of choice. If you want to use the entire pineapple for this recipe, then adjust the sweetener and coconut milk to the right amount.

4. Take your mold and sprinkle a bit of dried coconut at the top. Then pour in half an inch of popsicle mixture, sprinkle more coconut, add more mixture, and repeat until the mold is filled.

5. You can simply mix the dried coconut in if you'd prefer but the layers give it a fun design.

6. Add the stick and freeze for at least five hours.

7. These will last several weeks in the freezer.

Chapter 10 - Following the Alkaline Diet

Developing the eating habits of the people from the Alkaline region might be difficult if you don't follow proper guidelines. Now that you have the complete picture in your mind, it will not be hard. Often, beginners give up halfway because they assume that the diet isn't helpful. However, the Alkaline diet has been proven to be the best diet because of its many health benefits, including weight loss. If you are not witnessing positive results, it's because you have not followed the diet properly or you have not dedicated enough of your time to it. Unlike other diets, the Alkaline diet will take some time and you have to be consistent in following the diet if you want to see positive results. Furthermore, if you can follow these following tips, I promise you will succeed with this diet.

Consider eating whole grains: Consider grains such as brown rice, quinoa, popcorn, oatmeal, etc. These whole grain products can easily be purchased from your local grocery store. Pro tip: check for the word "whole" on the label when purchasing whole grain products.

Healthy portions: It is essential to consider healthy portions because this will determine whether you gain or lose weight. If you want to see positive results from the Alkaline diet, you must make sure you consume healthy portions. Also, enjoy the food you consume.

Savor your food: Most of us don't practice mindful eating but it is one of the essential aspects of eating. It is crucial you become mindful when eating. If you are eating for the sake of eating, is there a point in eating in the first place? There is no meaning in eating if you are not actually tasting the food. You should enjoy every bite that you take and you really taste the textures and flavors. You should take time to appreciate the food that is on your plate.

Kitchen tools and equipment needed: If you don't have the right kitchen tools and equipment, you will not be able to properly meal prep. If you don't properly meal prep, you will not be able to successfully complete this diet. The Alkaline diet is considered one of the most suitable diets for busy people. Hence, you must have the essential tools and equipment ready if you want to get the most out of this diet.

Set attainable expectations: If you are following the Alkaline diet intending to lose weight, you should be consistent in following the diet. You should not attempt to do something that will generate quick results. The moment you set unattainable expectations, you lose. It is important to focus your efforts on creating attainable expectations because only then you will be able to achieve your weight loss goals.

Don't store unhealthy foods: If you like junk food, it's time to give it up. Before you begin this diet, it's important you do something about all the junk food you have. The moment you get rid of it all, you will no longer be tempted to eat it when you feel bored or have cravings. It will be impossible to control your temptations and cravings if you know that junk food is readily available in your pantry, and only a few steps away from all your healthy food.

Eat with someone: The Alkaline diet encourages you to eat with friends and family because it helps increase your overall health. By socializing, you get the chance to enjoy the food that you are eating while also enjoying the time you spend with your family and friends.

Focus on motivations: Feeling motivated is crucial for anyone who's following a new diet because too often do people give up. To avoid giving up too early, begin by writing the reasons why you plan to follow the diet in the first place. Whenever you feel like giving up, you can go back and read the reasons that you wrote down. They can serve as a motivation for you to continue.

Forgive yourself: Don't be hard on yourself when times get tough. There will be times when you fall off track, and resort to eating unhealthy foods. That's okay. Forgive yourself and give yourself the time you need to get back on the right track.

Carry snacks with you: If you don't carry healthy snacks around with you, it will be hard for you to stick to the Alkaline diet. It is better to carry healthy snacks with you so that you don't resort to unhealthy ones.

FAQs and Facts of the Alkaline Diet
Can I eat carbs on a diet?
You may be wondering whether you can eat carbs while on the Alkaline diet. Well, carbs are not 100% unhealthy. In fact, your body needs carbs to create energy. So, what's so bad about them? Highly processed carbs are bad for your health. Also, what's unhealthy is the portion of carbs you consume. If you do not think about the portions you are eating, chances are you'll regain all the weight you just lost. That being said, you shouldn't give up on carbs entirely; instead, focus on healthy carbs and healthy portions.

Can I lose weight with this diet?
Of course! Many studies have shown the benefit of weight loss from the Alkaline diet. Even though the primary reason of the diet program was not for weight-loss, it has become a popular solution for weight-loss. The eating patterns followed by the people in the Alkaline region is healthy, therefore, it is just one of the reasons why you can lose weight by following this diet. There are a number of other reasons for why this diet helps with weight loss.

How do I shop for ingredients?
Some essential items to always have on your grocery list includes olive oil, seasonal vegetables, healthy grains, beans, and fish. You

should also consider buying your ingredients in bulk. That way, you can save money and simply store the food away and get it when you really need it. Before you shop for ingredients, review your weekly or daily meal plan so you don't buy items you won't need for that week or day.

How do I succeed on this diet?
It takes some time to enjoy all the benefits of the Alkaline diet. You might only witness changes in your weight after two weeks or more. If you understood the importance of the Alkaline diet from earlier, you will be ready to follow it even though it requires a lot of patience and hard work. If you want to succeed with this diet, you should be prepared to work hard.

Is the Alkaline diet easy to follow?
It is not an easy diet to follow but it is not complex either. This diet provides a lot of flexibility in regard to the types of food you can eat. There is no definite meal plan that you should follow. You can create your own or follow a plan that was created by someone else. However, the idea of planning for some dieters might be daunting. Some people don't like to make plans themselves, therefore, this diet can be harder for these people to follow.

Is exercising important?
Absolutely! However, you don't have to sign up for a gym membership to get in the exercise you need. Instead, become an active individual. One way you can do this is by commuting to work on your bicycle instead of taking your car to work. Or, you can engage in a morning walk before heading to work. If you don't like any of those suggestions, you can consider dancing or try a new sport. Remaining active is important because it keeps you healthy.

Is wine compulsory?

No, it is optional. If you don't like to drink wine, you don't need to include it in your diet.

Chapter 11 - Tasty Alkaline Recipes

Breakfast Recipes

Tomato, Cucumber and Feta Salad

Time needed: 10 minutes
Servings: 4

This is an ideal Alkaline salad that is enriched with a lot of flavor. This delicious dish can be prepared in as short as 10 minutes. You can also serve this dish with some grilled fish.

Ingredients

- 1 ½ tablespoon red-wine vinegar
- 1 teaspoon fresh oregano (chopped)
- Oregano leaves (for garnish)
- ½ teaspoon Dijon mustard
- ¼ teaspoon Kosher salt
- 3 tablespoons Extra-virgin olive oil
- 4 sliced crosswise Persian cucumber
- 2 cups (8 ounces) Campari tomatoes (wedges)
- 1 ½ ounce Feta cheese (crumbled)

How to Prepare

1. Take a medium-size bowl.

2. Whisk oregano, vinegar, salt, and mustard together.

3. Drizzle olive oil and whisk steadily.

4. Then, add cucumbers, feta cheese, tomatoes, and mix.

5. If preferred, garnish using the small oregano leaves.

6. For better taste, serve right away.

Recipe Notes

- If you can't find Persian cucumber and Campari tomatoes, you can opt for any other cucumbers or tomatoes, but note that there will be changes in the macros.
- If you are meal prepping, prepare the dressing ahead, transfer it to an airtight container, and refrigerate it so that you can use it when you are prepared to eat.
- You can refrigerate this dish for up to three days.

Avocado and Apple Smoothie

Time needed: 15 minutes
Servings: 2

Smoothies are a great go-to breakfast option for busy individuals. Green smoothies are not only delicious but also healthy! This breakfast will detoxify your body, and will make you feel great.

Ingredients

- 1 cup unsweetened almond milk
- 4 cups spinach
- 1 medium apple (peeled and quartered)
- 1 avocado (peeled and pitted)
- 1 banana (cut into chunks and frozen)
- 2 teaspoons honey

- ½ teaspoon ground ginger
- Ice cubes
- Almond butter, flaxseed, or chia seeds (optional)

How to Prepare

1. Take a high-powered blender.
2. Add almond milk, avocado, spinach, apples, honey, banana, ginger, ice cubes, and honey.
3. Blend the ingredients until smooth.
4. Taste and add spices and sweetness if needed.
5. Enjoy right away.

Recipe Notes

- You can store the leftovers in an airtight container and refrigerate them for a day. Or you can halve the ingredients if the smoothie is for one person.
- If you don't own a high-powered blender, you should blend the spinach, avocado, and almond milk separately first. Then, add banana, apple, ginger, and honey.
- Once you get a smooth texture, add ice cubes.

Cucumber and Heirloom Tomato Toast

Time needed: 5 minutes
Servings: 1

Find the freshest and ripest ingredients to prepare this toast and make it a delicious meal. You can make this dish in just five minutes, and it can be considered a great breakfast, dinner, or lunch meal; the choice is yours!

Ingredients

- 1 small heirloom tomato (diced)
- 1 Persian cucumber (diced)
- Pinch of oregano (dried)
- 1 teaspoon Extra-virgin oil
- 2 teaspoons whipped cream cheese (low-fat)
- 2 pieces whole grain bread
- 1 teaspoon balsamic glaze
- Black pepper and kosher salt

How to Prepare

1. Take a medium bowl.

2. Add in cucumber, tomato, oregano, olive oil and toss.

3. Then, season with black pepper and kosher salt.

4. Apply the cream cheese on the whole grain bread and add the salad on top with some balsamic glaze.

Lunch Recipes

Grilled Halloumi, Herbs, and Tomato Salad

Time needed: 10 minutes
Servings: 4

Normally this salad is made with grilled steak but with this recipe you can try it out with some grilled halloumi instead. This delicious and easy to make meal can be made in just 10 minutes.

Ingredients

- 1 pound tomatoes (sliced in circular shapes)
- ½ pound Halloumi cheese (four slabs)
- ½ lemon
- Extra-virgin olive oil (as needed)
- 5 basil leaves (torn)
- 2 tablespoons parsley leaves (finely chopped)
- Ground pepper and kosher salt

How to Prepare

1. Begin by preheating the grill and setting it to medium-high.

2. Next, place the tomatoes on four plates and squeeze the lemon over them. Also, season with ground pepper and kosher salt.

3. Once the grill is oiled, place the halloumi and let it cook. Make sure to flip sides and ensure it's cooked properly.

4. Spend around 1 minute on each side of the halloumi, or until you notice grill marks.

5. Place the finished halloumi on top of the neatly arranged tomatoes, drizzle olive oil and add parsley and basil.

6. Enjoy!

Toasted Za'atar Pita Bread with Mezze Plate

Time needed: 15 minutes
Servings: 2

This recipe is as exciting as its name. There's no doubt that you'll keep wanting more of this dish. The delicious herbed pitas are what make this dish so wonderful. Moreover, no cooking is required to prepare this recipe.

Ingredients

- 4 rounds whole-wheat pita
- 4 teaspoons za'atar
- 4 tablespoons extra-virgin olive oil
- 1 cup Greek yogurt
- 1 cup hummus
- 1 cup marinated artichoke hearts
- 1 cup red peppers (sliced and roasted)
- 2 cups cherry tomatoes
- 2 cups assorted olives
- 4 ounces salami
- Kosher salt and black pepper

How to Prepare

1. Take a large skillet and place it on medium-high heat.

2. Add olive oil to either side of the pitas and drizzle with za'atar.

3. Cook in batches.

4. Place pitas on the heated skillet and let it toast for about 2 minutes on each side.

5. Then, quarter each pita.

6. Next, sprinkle some pepper and salt on the Greek yogurt.

7. Finally, assemble your dish by dividing the pitas, hummus, artichoke hearts, Greek yogurt, olives, red peppers, salami, and tomatoes onto four plates.

The Cold Lemon Zucchini

Time needed: 20 minutes
Servings: 4

This dish is an enjoyable cold meal. This dish gives you the option to have something cold on days where the heat is too much to handle. This recipe is simple to prepare.

Ingredients

- 1 lemon (zested and juiced)
- ½ teaspoon Dijon mustard
- ½ teaspoon garlic powder
- ⅓ cup Olive oil
- 1 bunch radishes (thinly sliced)
- 1 tablespoon fresh thyme (chopped)
- 3 medium zucchinis (cut into noodles)
- Kosher salt and black pepper

How to Prepare

1. Take a bowl and whisk the lemon juice and zest, garlic powder, and mustard together.

2. Slowly, add olive oil and mix. Season with pepper and salt.

3. Meanwhile, take a large bowl and add the radishes and zucchini noodles. Then, add the prepared dressing. Make sure to toss until well coated.

4. Enjoy immediately by garnishing with thyme.

Roasted Red Pepper Sauce and Alkaline Quinoa Dish

Time needed: 20 minutes
Servings: 8

It's time to wave goodbye to time-consuming meal preparations. This lunch recipe is a special one. It's also a great recipe for holiday parties. You'll be saving a lot of time and energy preparing this dish. It only takes 20 minutes to prepare it.

Ingredients for the bowls

- Quinoa (cooked)
- Feta cheese
- Cucumber, spinach, or kale
- Kalamata olives
- Red onion (thinly sliced)
- Pepperoncini
- Hummus
- Parsley or fresh basil
- Salt, pepper, lemon juice, and olive oil

Ingredients roasted red pepper sauce

- ½ cup Olive oil
- 1 garlic clove
- ½ cup almonds
- 1 16 ounce jar roasted red peppers (drained)
- ½ teaspoon salt
- 1 lemon (juiced)

How to Prepare

1. With a blender of food processor, add all the ingredients needed to prepare the sauce. Pulse it until you get a thick texture.

2. To prepare the quinoa, read the instructions on the package. Once done, arrange the Alkaline quinoa bowl to your preference.

3. Enjoy with the prepared sauce.

Recipe Notes

- To cook the quinoa, you can use a rice cooker while you prepare everything else.
- If you are a vegetarian, you can exchange the feta cheese for white beans.
- Use plastic containers to store away any leftovers.

Salad Recipes

Avocado Dressing added Chickpea-and Kale Grain Bowl

Time needed: 20 minutes
Servings: 4

This particular salad bowl is filled with a number of colorful and flavorful ingredients. All the ingredients together will make it a great bowl; however, it's the avocado dressing which will add the final touch to it. It will not only add color to your salad but also a number of health benefits. This veggie bowl will help with digestion, and provide you with energy throughout the day. This is one of the best Alkaline salads that you can prepare in a short time.

Ingredients

- 1 cup boiling water
- ½ cup uncooked bulgur
- 1 ½ tablespoons olive oil
- 2 cans (15 ounces) chickpeas (unsalted, rinsed, and drained)
- 2 cups carrots (finely chopped)
- ½ cup shallots (vertically sliced)
- 4 cups lacinato kale (chopped)
- ½ cup parsley leaves (flat-leaf)
- ½ avocado (peeled and pitted)
- 1 garlic clove
- 1 tablespoon tahini (sesame seed paste)
- ½ teaspoon black pepper
- ¾ teaspoon Kosher salt
- 2 tablespoons extra-virgin olive oil
- 1 tablespoon lemon juice
- 1 tablespoon water
- ¼ teaspoon ground turmeric

How to Prepare

1. Take a medium-sized bowl and add in the bulgur and boiling water. Mix together for 10 minutes and drain.

2. Using paper towels, dry the chickpeas.

3. Meanwhile, place a skillet over high heat and add the olive oil.

4. Then, add carrots and chickpeas to the skillet and cook. Make sure to stir often. Let it cook for 6 minutes.

5. Add kale and cover the skillet. Wait around 2 minutes, or until wilted.

6. Stir chickpea mixture, parsley, shallots, pepper, and salt to the prepared bulgur and mix.

7. To make the avocado dressing, in a food processor, add olive oil, water, lemon juice, garlic, tahini, turmeric, and remaining salt.

8. Process until you get the smooth texture.

9. Divide bulgur equally among four bowls and drizzle the avocado mixture over top.

Pasta Salad with Eggplant and Tomatoes

Time needed: 20 minutes
Servings: 4

This is a filling salad that will leave you feeling satiated. It's normally not easy to feel satiated with just a bowl of salad but this one is an exception because of its filling and delicious ingredients.

Ingredients

- 8 ounces uncooked casarecce
- 1 tablespoon olive oil
- 2 cups eggplant (chopped)
- ¼ cup dry white wine
- 1 tablespoon garlic (minced)
- 2 pints cherry tomatoes (halved)
- 2 teaspoons white wine vinegar
- 2 teaspoons fresh thyme (chopped)
- ½ teaspoon Kosher salt
- 6 ounces burrata
- ½ teaspoon black pepper

How to Prepare

1. Read the directions on the package and cook the pasta accordingly.

2. In the last 3 minutes, add beans to the pasta. Drain the pasta and set aside a cup of cooking liquid from the pasta.

3. Meanwhile, take a large skillet and place it over medium-high heat.

4. Stir in eggplant and cook while stirring occasionally. Stir for around 4-5 minutes until tender.

5. Stir in garlic and cook for 1 minute, then, stir in half of the cherry tomatoes. Cook for about 2-3 minutes.

6. Next, add the wine and stir.

7. Stir in beans and pasta. Mix well. Now, add in a tablespoon of the cooking liquid you set aside.

8. Add the remaining tomatoes, salt, and vinegar.

9. Take four bowls and serve the pasta into the bowls.

10. Top with thyme, pepper, and burrata.

Recipe Notes

- If you don't have burrata, you can add 6 ounces of mozzarella and chop it into bite size pieces.

Snack Recipes

Carrot Cake Bites

Time needed: 15 minutes
Servings: 30-40 (varies as per the size you make)

Carrot cake bites are the best when you want something to snack on. This little snacks are so delicious that you might never stop snacking on them.

Ingredients

- 1 medium carrot (peeled and chopped)
- ½ cup almond butter
- ½ cup pure maple syrup
- 2 cups unsweetened flaked coconut
- 2 cups old fashioned oats
- ½ teaspoon vanilla
- ½ teaspoon Kosher salt
- 1 teaspoon cinnamon
- Chocolate chips (optional)

How to Prepare

1. Begin by cutting the carrot into chunks and then, add the chunks to a food processor. Pulse until chopped.

2. Keep aside chopped carrots, and add the coconut and oats. Pulse until chopped.

3. Then, add all the ingredients together and pulse until smooth. Use a spatula to combine all the ingredients if they stick to the processor bowl.

4. Add in chocolate chips; pulse once again.

5. Now, you can prepare the balls and freeze.

Quick Vegan Yogurt

Time needed: 5 minutes
Servings: 4

Homemade anything is always fun, and so is this homemade yogurt! Prepare this vegan yogurt with just three ingredients while sweetening it naturally.

Ingredients

- ½ cup cashews
- 2 cups frozen peaches
- 12 ounces tofu
- 1 tablespoon lemon juice
- ¼ cup liquid sweetener (agave, maple syrup, honey)
- 1 probiotic capsule (optional)

How to Prepare

1. Add all the ingredients together and blend on high speed. Blend until smooth.

2. Enjoy!

Recipe Notes

- You can store this yogurt in the fridge for up to 5 days.
- If you find it hard to blend the ingredients together, you can add ¼-½ cup of non-dairy milk. To blend easily, thaw frozen peaches first.

- If you want the probiotic boost, you can add a probiotic capsule to the mixture. Remove the cover and add the powder to the mixture. Adding the probiotic capsule is always optional.

Two-Minute Avocado Dip

Time needed: 2 minutes
Servings: 2

Avocado dip goes well with almost any variety of chips. Plus, it's also healthy. You can prepare avocado dip in as little as two minutes!

Ingredients

- 1 avocado
- ¼ cup plain Greek yogurt
- Lime juice to taste
- ¼ teaspoon salt
- Pinch of garlic powder

How to Prepare

1. Begin by mashing the avocado.

2. Add in the lime juice, yogurt, salt, and garlic powder.

3. Taste and adjust accordingly! Yes, simple as that.

Recipe Notes

- Add chopped cilantro if you wish, or add cayenne or jalapeno to spice it up.
- Dinner Recipes

Sweet Potato Noodles and Almond Sauce

Time needed: 20 minutes
Servings: 4

If you have been looking for delicious vegan dinner recipes for a while now, this is one of them. This recipe is filling and full of texture. It's also packed with a number of vitamins and proteins, making it a healthy meal.

Ingredients for Almond sauce

- 2 tablespoons extra-virgin olive oil
- 3 shallots (minced)
- 2 garlic cloves (minced)
- 2 cups unsweetened almond milk
- 3 tablespoons all-purpose flour
- 2 tablespoons Dijon mustard
- Salt and black pepper

Ingredients for Sweet potato noodles

- 2 tablespoons extra-virgin olive oil
- 3 sweet potatoes (cut into noodles)
- 4 cups torn kale
- ½ cup almonds (toasted and chopped)
- Salt and black pepper

How to Prepare

1. Begin by making the almond sauce. Take a medium-sized pot, add olive oil and place over medium heat.

2. Stir in garlic and shallots; sauté for one minute.

3. Add flour and cook for one minute.

4. Next, pour almond milk and mix to avoid lumps. Let it simmer for 4-5 minutes.

5. Add Dijon mustard and flavor the almond sauce with pepper and salt. Cover and reduce the heat.

6. Use a spiralizer to make noodles out of the sweet potatoes.

7. Take a large pan, add olive oil, and place it over medium heat.

8. Then, add in the noodles and stir occasionally. Wait 4-5 minutes or until tender.

9. Toss in the kale and sauce. Make sure the noodles are well coated.

10. Season the mixture with pepper and salt.

11. Add the almonds and serve.

Courgette, Shaved Fennel, and Orange Salad

Time needed: 15 minutes
Servings: 4

It's always enjoyable to eat a fresh salad. This recipe might be one of the most straightforward recipes for a salad you will ever make.

Ingredients

- 1 orange
- 2 small fennel bulbs
- 1 baby gem lettuce (washed and leaves separated)
- 2 small courgettes (green or yellow)
- 2 teaspoons sherry vinegar
- 4 tablespoons olive oil
- ½ cup lemon juice

How to Prepare

1. Peel the orange.

2. Cut the slices of the orange into halves. You can keep the juice collected from the orange as dressing.

3. Take a bowl and stir all the ingredients together.

4. Clean the fennel thoroughly, halve it, and cut the cores out. Then, slice the fennel into thin pieces.

5. Cut the ends of the courgettes with the help of a peeler.

6. Add in the orange juice that you kept aside, olive oil, and sherry vinegar to the same bowl.

7. Toss the mixture together so that everything combines well.

8. Before serving, add the mixed courgette, lettuce leaves, fennel, and orange slices together.

Mango Pineapple Salsa with Cajun Mahi Mahi

Time needed: 15 minutes
Servings: 4

This recipe is different from the rest. It is also probably a recipe you wouldn't normally make. I can assure you though that you will love its taste. The pineapple salsa makes this recipe that much better.

Ingredients for Cajun Mahi Mahi

- 1.5 pound of fresh Mahi Mahi fillets
- 1 tablespoon Cajun spice seasoning
- ½ tablespoon garlic powder
- 2 tablespoons grapeseed oil

Ingredients Mango Pineapple Salsa

- 1 mango (finely diced)
- 1 cup pineapple (fresh diced)
- ¼ cup red onion (finely diced)
- ¼ cup fresh cilantro (chopped)
- 1-2 tablespoons lime juice
- Kosher salt

How to Prepare

1. Take a small bowl and add the mango, fresh cilantro, pineapple, salt, and lime juice. Mix everything and keep it aside.

2. In another bowl, add in cajun spice and garlic powder and mix.

3. Dry the Mahi Mahi fillets.

4. Season the Mahi Mahi fillets using cajun seasoning mixture.

5. Heat a skillet to medium-high heat. Then, heat the grapeseed oil.

6. Sear the Mahi Mahi fillets for 2-3 minutes on each side.

7. Remove from the stove and let it sit for a minute.

8. Enjoy!

Cauliflower Rice

Time needed: 20 minutes
Servings: 4

This recipe is similar to fried rice, only it is a much healthier alternative.

Ingredients

- 5 cups (24 ounces) cauliflower florets
- 2 tablespoons of reduced sodium soy sauce
- 1 tablespoon sesame oil
- 1 tablespoon ginger (grated)
- 2 tablespoons vegetable oil
- 2 green onions (thinly sliced)
- ¼ teaspoon white pepper
- 6 ounces broccoli florets (chopped)
- 2 garlic cloves (minced)
- 1 onion (diced)
- 2 carrots (peeled and grated)
- ½ cup frozen peas
- ½ cup frozen corn
- ½ teaspoon sesame seeds

How to Prepare

1. Before making the cauliflower rice, you must use a food processor to pulse the cauliflower so that it turns into rice. Pulse it for around 3 minutes and set aside.

2. Take a bowl and whisk the sesame oil, soy sauce, white pepper, ginger, and place it aside.

3. Then, take a medium-sized skillet and heat a tablespoon of oil and set it to low heat.

4. Next, add the remaining oil to the skillet and place over medium-high heat. Add onion and garlic to it and occasionally stir. Cook for 3-4 minutes. Add corn, carrots, broccoli, and peas and stir occasionally. Wait 3-4 minutes, or until vegetables are tender.

5. Add cauliflower, soy sauce, and green onions. Cook for 4 minutes while stirring occasionally, until cauliflower is tender.

6. Garnish the finished product with sesame seeds and serve.

The Alkaline diet comes with many benefits. However, what turns many people away is that they will be limited in terms of meal intake. We have provided various forms of Alkaline diet recipes in this manual. Hence, you can get creative and play around with it.

Besides, the Alkaline diet lifestyle does not have to be a burden or a restriction. The aim of going into Alkaline diet for many people is to lose weight and enjoy the many health benefits that come along with it. Hence, be sure to follow all you have learned in this book and be creative about how you eat. Diet plan gets boring, and many people find it difficult to stick with it when are restricted to tasteless meals.

Be sure to get your house in order in preparation for the Alkaline diet lifestyle journey. Get rid of every food that is not Alkaline diet friendly. If possible, ask your spouse or any of your housemates to join you in the diet. It gets easier if you are not alone. Besides, the absence of Alkaline diet friendly food also removed the temptation of going above your daily carb limit.

While Alkaline diet comes with a whole lot of health benefits, users need to be aware of the potential danger. We have listed some class of people not fit for the diet. Besides, if you are on any medication, be sure to talk to your doctor before starting the Alkaline diet. In addition to that, be prepared mentally for the side effects known as Alkaline diet flu. The good news, however, is that you can lessen the side effect of transition into Alkaline diet by drinking a lot of water, this is not negotiable.

While the majority of food classes you will concentrate on is fats, be aware that there are good fats and bad fats. Hence, be sure to follow all the recommended ideas in this manual. We have listed bad fats you should stay away from. Keep them in mind, so they do not sabotage your effort to get into Alkaline diet.

On a final note, be aware that you will not likely have the same result with other people, even your spouse if you follow the Alkaline diet together. Keep this in mind and do not be discouraged. The reason for this is due to the many variables present. Your body, your activity level, and your ages differ. The way you workout and the kind of lifestyle you lead all add to the variables. Be sure to stick to the plan and be faithful with it. When you get to Alkaline diet, you will experience the tremendous health benefits of the Alkaline diet.

Some More Alkaline diet Recipes

Coconut Alkaline Diet Coffee

Ingredients
- Ghee – 1 tablespoon
- Coconut oil – half tablespoon
- Black coffee – 1 cup

How to Prepare

Put all the ingredients in a blender and blend thoroughly

Alkaline Diet Frittata

List of Ingredients
- Baby Spinach – 4 ounces
- Shredded cheddar cheese – 1 cup
- Sliced mushroom – 1 cup
- Butter – 2 tablespoons
- Pepper – 2 tablespoons
- Salt – half teaspoon
- Heavy cream – a quarter of a cup

How to Prepare
1. Preheat your over to 1800 degrees.
2. Over the high heat, place a cast iron, preferably frying pan.
3. Leave for about four minutes and add butter.
4. Get your sliced mushroom ready and pour in the pan.
5. Sauté the entire mixture for about three minutes.
6. Into the cooking mixture, add spinach and cook for two more minutes till it is wilted.
7. Remove from the heat and add some cheddar cheese into the pan.
8. Get a mixing bowl. Put in cream, pepper, and salt.
9. Whisk the entire mixture thoroughly till it is combines.
10. Pour all the mixture into the pan and place in the oven.

11. Bake for 20 minutes.

12. After this, it is ready for serving.

White Lasagna Stuffed Peppers

List of Ingredients
- Sweet pepper – 2 large, seeded and halved
- Garlic salt - 1 tablespoon
- Ground turkey – 12 ounces
- Mozzarella – 1 cup
- Ricotta Cheese – 1 cup
- Cherry tomato – 8 (optional though)

How to Prepare
1. Raise your over to temperature as high as 205-degrees Centigrade.

2. Put the halved sweet pepper into the baking dish and spread one quarter garlic salt in it.

3. Unto the pepper, spread out the turkey. Sprinkle another quarter teaspoon of garlic salt.

4. Place the mixture in the oven and bake for about 30 minutes.

5. Into the pepper, sprinkle the ricotta cheese and the mozzarella and the remaining garlic salt.

6. If you are using the tomato, slice it into the mixture.

7. Bake for half an hour till the meat is well cooked, the pepper softens out, and the cheese becomes golden.

8. Serve into four plates and enjoy.

Fresh Bell Pepper Basil Pizza

List of Ingredients for the Pizza base
- Mozzarella Cheese – 6 ounces
- Almond flour – half cup
- Psyllium husk powder – 2 tablespoons
- Italian seasoning – 1 teaspoon
- Parmesan Cheese – 2 tablespoons
- Salt – half teaspoon
- Pepper – half teaspoon

List of Ingredients for the toppings
- Shredded cheddar cheeses – 4 ounces
- Tomato – a piece
- Marinara sauce – a quarter of a cup
- Bell pepper – two third
- Basil – 3 tablespoons

How to Prepare
1. Preheat your oven to a temperature of 204 degrees Centigrade.

2. Put the Mozzarella cheese in your microwave till it is melted.

3. Put all the pizza base ingredients in the cheese and mix thoroughly.

4. With a rolling pin, flatten the dough into a circle.

5. Put the entire mixture in the oven for 10 minutes.

6. Get it out of the oven and spread the topping ingredient on top.

7. Put it back in the oven and allow it to bake for an extra 10 minutes.

Brownie Batter Mug Cake

List of Ingredients
- Almond flour – 1 tablespoon
- Flaxseed meal – 1 tablespoon
- Butter – 2 tablespoons
- Baking powder – half teaspoon
- Cocoa powder – 1 tablespoon
- Brownie Batter Almond Butter – one and a half tablespoon

How to Prepare
1. Put the entire ingredient in a mug and mix.

2. Microwave for about a minute.

3. Leave it to cool and pour the content in a plate, leaving the mug upside down.

4. To make the brownie flow out, tap the mug and enjoy.

Low Carb Cheesecake Brownies

List of Ingredients for the brownie
- Salt – half teaspoon
- Almond flour – three quarter cup
- Erythritol – two-third of a cup
- Cocoa powder - two-third of a cup

List of Ingredients for the Cheesecake
- Vanilla extract – 1 teaspoon
- Erythritol – One-quarter of a cup
- Cream cheese – 8 ounces

How to Prepare
1. Preheat the oven to 175-degree centigrade.

2. With a parchment, line the bottom of an 8 by 8 pan.

3. Spray cooking spray on the pan.

4. Cream the sweetener and cream cheese together till it is smooth.

5. Add the vanilla and mix thoroughly till you achieve a cream and soft feeling.

6. Melt the butter, add sweetener, salt, and cocoa.

7. Stir vigorously till the sweetener dissolves.

8. Add the almond flour slowly as you mix till it forms a good dough.

9. Add two third of the brownie batter into your prepared pan.

10. Dollop your cheese batter into the brownie.

11. Pour the rest of the brownie batter.

12. Bake for like 23 minutes and keep an eye on it.

13. Allow to cook and cut.

14. Refrigerate it for about 10 minutes.

15. It can be left in a refrigerator for 3 days.

Loaded Cauliflower Mashed Potatoes

List of Ingredients
- Cauliflower – 1 head
- Garlic – 1 clove
- Butter – 3 tablespoons
- Salt – half teaspoon
- Pepper – one eight teaspoons
- Green onions
- Sour cream – 1 tablespoon

How to Prepare
1. Heat a pot of water to boiling point and put the cauliflower in.

2. Reduce the heat and simmer for an average of 10 minutes.

3. Drain the water from the cauliflower.

4. Get a food processor, add the garlic, pepper, salt, cauliflower, and sour cream.

5. Process the entire mixture for about two minutes.

6. Spread some cheese, green onions and crumbles on the top.

7. It is best served warm.

~ For us, people's health is fundamental, which is why we decided to create this essential guide. We hope with all our heart that you enjoyed it and we hope you can recommend it to your friends or loved ones ~

Because being healthy is everyone's right.

THANK YOU

Copyright © 2019 Emma Jason

All rights reserved.